Free Video  **Free Video**

Essential Test Tips Video from Trivium Test Prep

Dear Customer,

Thank you for purchasing from Trivium Test Prep! We're honored to help you prepare for your exam.

To show our appreciation, we're offering a **FREE** *KNAT Essential Test Tips* **Video by Trivium Test Prep.*** Our video includes 35 test preparation strategies that will make you successful on your big exam. All we ask is that you email us your feedback and describe your experience with our product. Amazing, awful, or just so-so: we want to hear what you have to say!

To receive your **FREE** *KNAT Essential Test Tips* **Video**, please email us at 5star@triviumtestprep.com. Include "Free 5 Star" in the subject line and the following information in your email:

1. The title of the product you purchased.
2. Your rating from 1 – 5 (with 5 being the best).
3. Your feedback about the product, including how our materials helped you meet your goals and ways in which we can improve our products.
4. Your full name and shipping address so we can send your **FREE** *KNAT Essential Test Tips* **Video**.

If you have any questions or concerns please feel free to contact us directly at 5star@triviumtestprep.com.

Thank you!

– Trivium Test Prep Team

*To get access to the free video please email us at 5star@triviumtestprep.com, and please follow the instructions above.

KAPLAN NURSING SCHOOL ENTRANCE EXAM STUDY GUIDE

KNAT Exam Prep Book with Practice Test Questions

TABLE OF CONTENTS

ONLINE RESOURCES

To help you fully prepare for your KNAT, Ascencia Test Prep includes online resources with the purchase of this study guide.

PRACTICE TESTS

In addition to the practice test included in this book, we also offer an online exam. Since many exams today are computer based, getting to practice your test-taking skills on the computer is a great way to prepare.

FLASH CARDS

A convenient supplement to this study guide, Ascencia's flash cards enable you to review important terms easily on your computer or smartphone.

CHEAT SHEETS

Review the core skills you need to master the exam with easy-to-read Cheat Sheets.

FROM STRESS TO SUCCESS

Watch "From Stress to Success," a brief but insightful YouTube video that offers the tips, tricks, and secrets experts use to score higher on the exam.

REVIEWS

Leave a review, send us helpful feedback, or sign up for Ascencia Test Prep promotions—including free books!

Access these materials at: **http://ascenciatestprep.com/knat-online-resources**

INTRODUCTION

The Kaplan Nursing School Admissions Test (KNAT) was developed by Kaplan for use by nursing programs during the application process. The exam evaluates candidates' relevant knowledge and skills so that they can be accurately placed in nursing education programs leading to RN licensure. The KNAT is also used to identify areas in reading, writing, math, and science where nursing students need remediation.

What's on the KNAT?

The KNAT is a multiple-choice test. It tests concepts in reading comprehension, writing, math, and science.

Test	Concepts	Number of Questions	Time
Reading Comprehension	main idea, supporting idea, inferences, details, interpreting information	22	45 minutes
Writing	grammar, mechanics, paragraph logic and development	21	45 minutes
Mathematics	arithmetic, fractions and decimals, ratios and proportions, units and measurements	28	45 minutes
Science	body systems (muscular, skeletal, nervous, renal/urinary, endocrine, circulatory, and respiratory), electrolytes and homeostasis	20	30 minutes
Total		**91 questions**	**2 hours and 45 minutes**

How is the KNAT Administered?

The KNAT is administered by individual health care education programs. Most programs will require you to create an account with Kaplan and to take the test at a specified testing location, usually on its campus. You should check with the program to which you are applying to find testing dates and locations. If you want to report your KNAT score to a school at which you did not test, you will need to contact the school's admissions office.

Before you take the KNAT, carefully check the policies and procedures for your particular test site. Fees and payment methods will vary by school. In addition, most schools will have specific requirements for what you will need to bring (e.g., identification, pencils) and what not to bring (e.g., calculators, cell phones).

The test will begin with a fifteen-minute tutorial that does not count toward the time limit for the exam.

Keep in mind that schools may require you to take the KNAT the same year that you are applying.

How is the KNAT Scored?

Scores are available immediately once you complete your exam. You may also access your scores through your Kaplan account.

You will receive a scaled percentage score ranging from 0 – 100 percent for each of the four sections of the exam and a cumulative percentage score reflecting your performance on the entire exam.

Minimum score requirements are determined by individual health care education programs. Check with your school to find out the minimum score required. Some schools require a cumulative score of 65 percent; others may require certain minimum scores on different sections.

Ascencia Test Prep

With health care fields such as nursing, pharmacy, emergency care, and physical therapy becoming the fastest-growing industries in the United States, individuals looking to enter the health care industry or rise in their field need high-quality, reliable resources. Ascencia Test Prep's study guides and test preparation materials are developed by credentialed industry professionals with years of experience in their respective fields. Ascencia recognizes that health care professionals nurture bodies and spirits, and save lives. Ascencia Test Prep's mission is to help health care workers grow.

ONE: READING

Reading Comprehension

On the KNAT, you must read nine short passages and answer twenty-two reading questions. You have forty-five minutes to complete this section.

Most passages will be about health or medicine. You do not need any outside knowledge to answer the questions.

Reading questions ask about reading comprehension skill: understanding the main idea of a passage, specific details, drawing inferences, and more. This section reviews different types of reading comprehension questions you will encounter.

THE MAIN IDEA

The **topic** is a word or short phrase that explains what a passage is about. The **main idea** is a complete sentence that explains what the author is trying to say about the topic. Generally, the **topic sentence** is the first (or near the first) sentence in a paragraph. It is a general statement that introduces the topic so that the reader knows what to expect.

The **summary sentence**, on the other hand, frequently (but not always!) comes at the end of a paragraph or passage because it wraps up all the ideas presented. This sentence summarizes what an author has said about the topic. Some passages, particularly short ones, will not include a summary sentence.

QUICK REVIEW

To find the main idea, identify the topic and then ask, "What is the author trying to tell me about the topic?"

Table 1.1. Identifying Topic and Main Idea

The cisco, a foot-long freshwater fish native to the Great Lakes, once thrived throughout the basin but had virtually disappeared by the 1950s. However, today fishermen are pulling them up by the net-load in Lake Michigan and Lake Ontario. It is highly unusual for a native species to revive, and the reason for the cisco's reemergence is even more unlikely. The cisco have an invasive species—quagga mussels—to thank for their return. Quagga mussels depleted nutrients in the lakes, harming other species highly dependent on these nutrients. Cisco, however, thrive in low-nutrient environments. As other species—many of which were invasive—diminished, cisco flourished in their place.

Table 1.1. Identifying Topic and Main Idea (continued)	
Topic sentence	The cisco, a foot-long freshwater fish native to the Great Lakes, once thrived throughout the basin but had virtually disappeared by the 1950s.
Topic	cisco
Summary sentence	As other species—many of which were invasive—diminished, cisco flourished in their place.
Main idea	Cisco had nearly disappeared from the lake, but now flourish thanks to the invasive quagga mussel.

PRACTICE QUESTIONS

1. Tourists flock to Yellowstone National Park each year to view the geysers that bubble and erupt throughout it. What most of these tourists do not know is that these geysers are formed by a caldera—a hot crater in the earth's crust—which was created by a series of three eruptions of an ancient super volcano. These eruptions, which began 2.1 million years ago, spewed between 1,000 to 2,450 cubic kilometers of volcanic matter at such a rate that the volcano's magma chamber collapsed, creating the craters.

   What is the topic of the passage?

   A) tourists

   B) geysers

   C) volcanic eruptions

   D) super volcanos

2. The Battle of Little Bighorn, commonly called Custer's Last Stand, was a battle between the Lakota, the Northern Cheyenne, the Arapaho, and the Seventh Cavalry Regiment of the US Army. Led by war leaders Crazy Horse and Chief Gall and the religious leader Sitting Bull, the allied tribes of the Plains Indians decisively defeated their US foes. Two hundred and sixty-eight US soldiers were killed, including General George Armstrong Custer, two of his brothers, his nephew, his brother-in-law, and six Indian scouts.

   What is the main idea of this passage?

   A) Most of General Custer's family died in the Battle of Little Bighorn.

   B) The Seventh Cavalry regiment was formed to fight Native American tribes.

   C) Sitting Bull and George Custer were fierce enemies.

   D) The Battle of Little Bighorn was a significant victory for the Plains Indians.

SUPPORTING DETAILS

Statements that describe or explain the main idea are **supporting details**. Supporting details are often found after the topic sentence. They support the main idea through examples, descriptions, and explanations.

HELPFUL HINT

To find supporting details, look for sentences that connect to the main idea and tell more about it.

Authors may add details to support their argument or claim. **Facts** are details that point to truths, while **opinions** are based on personal beliefs or judgments. To differentiate between fact and opinion, look for statements that express feelings, attitudes, or beliefs that can't be proven (opinions) and statements that can be proven (facts).

Table 1.2. Supporting Details and Fact and Opinion

Bait is an important element of fishing. Some people use live bait, such as worms and night crawlers. Others use artificial bait, such as lures and spinners. Live bait has a scent that fish are drawn to. Live bait is a good choice for fishing. It's cheap and easy to find. Lures can vibrate, make noise, and mimic the movements of some fish. People should choose artificial bait over live bait because it can be used multiple times.

Supporting details	Lures can vibrate, make noise, and mimic the movements of some fish.
Fact	Live bait has a scent that fish are drawn to.
Opinion	Live bait is a good choice for fishing.

PRACTICE QUESTIONS

3. Increasingly, companies are turning to subcontracting services rather than hiring full-time employees. This provides companies with advantages like greater flexibility, reduced legal responsibility to employees, and lower possibility of unionization within the company. However, this has led to increasing confusion and uncertainty over the legal definition of employment. Courts have grappled with questions about the hiring company's responsibility in maintaining fair labor practices. Companies argue that they delegate that authority to subcontractors, while unions and other worker advocate groups argue that companies still have a legal obligation to the workers who contribute to their business.

    Which detail BEST supports the idea that contracting employees is beneficial to companies?

    A) Uncertainty over the legal definition of employment increases.

    B) Companies still have a legal obligation to contractors.

    C) There is a lower possibility of unionization within the company.

    D) Contractors, not companies, control fair labor practices.

4. Chalk is a colorful way for kids and adults to have fun and be creative. Chalk is used on playgrounds and sidewalks. Children love to draw pictures in different colors. The designs are beautiful, but they are also messy. Chalk doesn't clean up easily. It has to wash away. Chalk is also used by cafés and bakeries. Shops use chalk to showcase their menus and special items. It is a great way to advertise their food.

    Which statement from the passage is an opinion?

    A) It is a great way to advertise their food.

    B) Chalk doesn't clean up easily.

    C) It has to wash away.

    D) Shops use chalk to showcase their menus and special items.

DRAWING CONCLUSIONS

Readers can use information that is **explicit**, or clearly stated, along with information that is **implicit**, or indirect, to make inferences and **draw conclusions**. Readers can determine meaning from what is implied by using details, context clues, and prior knowledge. When answering questions, consider what is known from personal

HELPFUL HINT

Look for facts, character actions and dialogue, how each sentence connects to the topic, and the author's reasoning for an argument when drawing conclusions.

experiences and make note of all information the author has provided before drawing a conclusion.

Table 1.3. Drawing Conclusions

When the Spanish-American War broke out in 1898, the US Army was small and under-staffed. President William McKinley called for 1,250 volunteers to serve in the First US Volunteer Calvary. The ranks were quickly filled by cowboys, gold prospectors, hunters, gamblers, Native Americans, veterans, police officers, and college students looking for an adventure. The officer corps was composed of veterans of previous wars. With more volunteers than it could accept, the army set high standards: all the recruits had to be skilled on horseback and with guns. Consequently, they became known as the Rough Riders.

Question	Why are the volunteers named Rough Riders?
Explicit information	different people volunteered, men were looking for adventure, recruits had to be extremely skilled on horseback and with guns due to a glut of volunteers
Implicit information	Men had previous occupations, officer corps veterans worked with volunteers.
Conclusion drawn	The men were called Rough Riders because they were inexperienced yet particularly enthusiastic to help with the war and were willing to put in extra effort to join.

PRACTICE QUESTION

5. After World War I, political and social forces pushed for a return to normalcy in the United States. The result was disengagement from the larger world and increased focus on American economic growth and personal enjoyment. Caught in the middle were American writers, raised on the values of the prewar world and frustrated with what they viewed as the superficiality and materialism of postwar American culture. Many of them fled to Paris, where they became known as the "lost generation," creating a trove of literary works criticizing their home culture and delving into their own feelings of alienation.

    Which conclusion about the effects of war is most likely true?

    A) War served as an inspiration for literary works.

    B) It was difficult to stabilize countries after war occurred.

    C) Writers were torn between supporting war and their own ideals.

    D) Individual responsibility and global awareness declined after the war.

THE AUTHOR'S PURPOSE AND POINT OF VIEW

The **author's purpose** is an author's reason for writing a text. Authors may write to share an experience, entertain, persuade, or inform readers. This can be done through persuasive, expository, and narrative writing.

Persuasive writing influences the actions and thoughts of readers. Authors state an opinion, then provide reasons that support the opinion. **Expository writing** outlines and explains steps in a process. Authors focus on a sequence of events. **Narrative writing** tells a story. Authors include a setting, plot, characters, problem, and solution in the text.

Authors also share their **point of view** (perspectives, attitudes, and beliefs) with readers. Identify the author's point of view by word choice, details, descriptions, and characters' actions. The author's attitude or **tone** can be found in word choice that conveys feelings or stance on a topic.

Text structure is the way the author organizes a text. A text can be organized to show problem and solution, comparison and contrast, or even cause and effect. Structure of a text can give insight into an author's purpose and point of view. If a text is organized to pose an argument or advertise a product, it can be considered persuasive. The author's point of view will be revealed in how thoughts and opinions are expressed in the text.

STUDY TIP
Use the acronym **P.I.E.S.**—*persuade*, *inform*, *entertain*, *state*—to help you remember elements of an author's purpose.

Table 1.4. The Author's Purpose and Point of View

Superfoods are foods that are found in nature. They contain rich nutrients and are low in calories. Many people are concerned about healthy diets and weight loss, so superfoods are a great meal choice! Rich antioxidants and vitamins found in superfoods decrease the risk of diseases and aid in heart health.

Author's purpose	persuade readers of the benefit of superfoods
Point of view	advocates superfoods as "a great meal choice"
Tone	positive, encouraging, pointing out the benefits of super-foods, using positive words like *great* and *rich*
Structure	cause and effect to show use of superfoods and results

PRACTICE QUESTIONS

6. University of California, Berkeley, researchers decided to tackle an age-old problem: why shoelaces come untied. They recorded the shoelaces of a volunteer walking on a treadmill by attaching devices to record the acceleration, or g-force, experienced by the knot. The results were surprising. A shoelace knot experiences more g-force from a person walking than any rollercoaster can generate. However, if the person simply stomped or swung their feet—the two movements that make up a walker's stride—the g-force was not enough to undo the knots.

What is the purpose of this passage?

A) to confirm if shoelaces always come undone

B) to compare the force of treadmills and rollercoasters

C) to persuade readers to tie their shoes tighter

D) to describe the results of an experiment on shoelaces

7. What do you do with plastic bottles? Do you throw them away, or do you recycle or reuse them? As landfills continue to fill up, there will eventually be no place to put our trash. If you recycle or reuse bottles, you will help reduce waste and turn something old into a creative masterpiece!

Which of the following BEST describes what the author believes?

A) Landfills are unnecessary.

B) Reusing objects requires creativity.

C) Recycling helps the environment.

D) Reusing objects is better than recycling.

8. Negative cinematic representations of gorillas have provoked fear and contribute to hunting practices that endanger gorilla populations. It's a shame that many films portray them as scary and aggressive creatures. Their size and features should not be cause for alarm. Gorillas are actually shy and act aggressively only when provoked.

   What can be inferred about the author's attitude toward gorillas?

   A) The author is surprised that people do not know the truth about gorillas.

   B) The author is concerned that movies distort people's opinion of gorillas.

   C) The author is saddened by the decrease in gorilla populations.

   D) The author is afraid that gorillas are being provoked.

9. Want smoother skin? Try *Face Lace*, a mix of shea butter and coconut oil. Like most creams, it's soft and easy to apply. We rank #1 in sales and free trials. Our competitor *Smooth Moves* may be great for blemishes, but we excel at reducing the signs of aging!

   What is the structure of this text?

   A) cause and effect

   B) order and sequence

   C) problem and solution

   D) compare and contrast

COMPARING PASSAGES

Sometimes readers need to compare and contrast two texts. After reading and identifying the main idea of each text, look for similarities and differences in the main idea, details, claims, evidence, characters, and so on.

When answering questions about two texts, first identify whether the question is about a similarity or a difference. Then look for specific details in the text that connect to the answers. After that, determine which answer choice best describes the similarity or difference.

HELPFUL HINT

Use a Venn diagram, table, or highlighters to organize similarities and differences between texts.

Table 1.5. Comparing Passages

Apple Cider Vinegar

Apple cider vinegar has many medicinal properties. It is used for cleaning and disinfecting. When ingested, it lowers blood sugar levels, increasing insulin function and fighting diabetes. Studies are being conducted to determine if it can aid in shrinking tumors and cancer cells, and lower the risk of heart disease.

Alkaline Water

Many people believe that alkaline water increases immune system support; prevents cancer; and aids in antiaging, detoxification, and weight loss. Unfortunately, having an excess amount of alkaline water in the body could produce nausea, vomiting, and tremors.

Similarities (comparison)	Both substances are ingested and used to fight diseases.
Differences (contrast)	Alkaline water has negative side effects, whereas apple cider vinegar is being studied to prove its usefulness.

10. Panda Bears

Panda bears live in China's bamboo forests. They eat bamboo and are excellent tree climbers. New roads and railroads break the flow of the forest, isolating panda populations. This decreases the amount of food pandas can access during the year.

Polar Bears

Polar bears live in the Arctic and are the largest land carnivores in the world. They eat seals and walruses. As the sea gets larger from melting ice, polar bears have to travel longer distances for food. Their thick white fur provides warmth and traction for their feet on the ice. They are good swimmers.

Which of these statements BEST compares the information in both texts?

A) A carnivore's diet depends on animals in the area.

B) The destruction of habitats affects food supply.

C) Animals must be able to move easily in their environment.

D) An animal's population can change its habitat.

MEANING OF WORDS

To understand the meanings of unfamiliar words, use **context clues**. Context clues are hints the author provides to help readers define difficult words. They can be found in words or phrases in the same sentence or in a neighboring sentence. Look for synonyms, antonyms, definitions, examples, and explanations in the text to determine the meaning of the unfamiliar word.

Sometimes parts of a word can make its meaning easier to determine. **Affixes** are added to **root words** (a word's basic form) to modify meaning. **Prefixes** are added to the beginning of root words, while **suffixes** are added to the ending. Divide words into parts, finding meaning in each part. Take, for example, the word *unjustifiable*: the prefix is *un–* (*not*), the root word is *justify* ("to prove reasonable"), and the suffix is *–able* (referring to a quality).

Another way to determine the meaning of unknown words is to consider their denotation and connotation with other words in the sentence. **Denotation** is the literal meaning of a word, while **connotation** is the positive or negative associations of a word.

Authors use words to convey thoughts, but the meaning may be different from a literal meaning of the words. This is called **figurative language**. Types of figurative language include similes, metaphors, hyperboles, and personification.

Similes compare two things that are not alike with the words *like* or *as*. Metaphors are used to compare two things that are not exactly alike but may share a certain characteristic.

Hyperboles are statements that exaggerate something in order to make a point or draw attention to a certain feature. Personification involves using human characteristics to describe an animal or object.

HELPFUL HINT

Use what you know about a word to figure out its meaning, then look for clues in the sentence or paragraph.

Table 1.6. Meanings of Words

Have you ever gone to a flea market? There are rows of furniture, clothing, and antiques waiting for discovery. Unlike a museum with items on display, flea markets are opportunities to learn and shop. Vendors bring their handmade goods to this communal event to show their crafts and make money.

Context clues	Vendors are people who sell things; people shop at a flea market.
Affixes	The prefix com– in communal means with or together.
Meaning	Communal means "shared with a community."

PRACTICE QUESTIONS

11. The Bastille, Paris's famous historical prison, was originally built in 1370 as a fortification—called a bastide in Old French—to protect the city from English invasion. It rose 100 feet into the air, had eight towers, and was surrounded by a moat more than eighty feet wide. In the seventeenth century, the government **converted** the fortress into an elite prison for upper-class felons, political disruptors, and spies.

    Which word or phrase can be used to determine the meaning of converted?

    A) originally built

    B) fortification

    C) felons

    D) historical prison

12. Breaking a world record is no easy feat. An application and video submission of an amazing skill may not be enough. Potential record breakers may need to demonstrate their skill in front of an official world records judge. The judge will watch a performance of a record attempt to determine if the record-breaking claim is **credible**. After all evidence is collected, reviewed, and approved, a certificate for the new world record is granted!

    Based on affixes and context clues, what does credible mean?

    A) believable

    B) achievable

    C) likeable

    D) noticeable

13. Every year people gather in Durham Park to participate in the Food Truck Rodeo. A band plays, and the food trucks are like a carnival of delicious treats. The aroma of food draws all who pass by, creating a large crowd. The event is free to attend; patrons pay only for what they want to eat. From pizzas and burgers to hotdogs and pastries, there's something for everyone!

    Which type of figurative language is used in the second sentence?

    A) hyperbole

    B) metaphor

    C) personification

    D) simile

RECOGNIZING SEQUENCES

Signal words indicate steps of a process, reveal a sequence of events, or show the **logic** of a passage. These words will tell you when things need to happen in a certain order. Signal words should show a transition from one event or step to another.

When reading a passage, you will find that signal words can be used to follow the direction of the author's ideas and the sequence of events. Signal words show time order and how details flow in a chronological way.

HELPFUL HINT

To find signal words, ask, "What happened first and what happened after that?"

Table 1.7. Following Directions and Recognizing Sequences

NASA wanted to launch a man from Earth to the moon. At first they used satellites for launch tests. Then in June of 1968, astronauts aboard the Apollo 8 launched into space and circled the moon ten times before returning to Earth. Finally, in 1969 three astronauts reached the moon in the Apollo 11 spacecraft. After a successful landing, two members of the crew walked on the moon. During their walk they collected data and samples of rocks. They returned as heroes of space exploration.	
Signal words	At first, then, finally, after, during

PRACTICE QUESTION

14. Babies learn to move their bodies over time. Head control is first developed at two months to create strong neck, back, and tummy muscles. Next, the abilities to reach, grasp, and sit up with support happen around four to six months. By the end of six months, babies learn to roll over. After six to nine months, babies can sit on their own and crawl. During age nine to twelve months, pulling and standing up are mastered. Finally, after gaining good balance, babies take their first steps!

Which BEST describes the order of a baby's movement over time?

A) roll over, control head, sit up, crawl

B) sit up, roll over, crawl, walk

C) control head, reach, crawl, roll over

D) sit up, grasp, crawl, walk

1. **B) is correct.** The topic of the passage is geysers. Tourists, volcanic eruptions, and super volcanos are all mentioned in the explanation of what geysers are and how they are formed.

2. **D) is correct.** The author writes that "the allied tribes...decisively defeated their US foes," and the remainder of the passage provides details to support this idea.

3. **C) is correct.** The passage specifically presents this detail as one of the advantages of subcontracting services.

4. **A) is correct.** The statement "It is a great way to advertise their food" is a judgment about how the shops use chalk to show menu items to customers. The word *great* expresses a feeling, and the idea cannot be proven.

5. **D) is correct.** After the war, there was a lack of focus on the world and greater focus on personal comforts, which writers viewed as superficiality and materialism.

6. **D) is correct.** The text provides details on the experiment as well as its results.

7. **C) is correct.** The author states that recycling and reusing objects reduces waste, which helps the environment.

8. **B) is correct.** The author demonstrates disapproval of film portrayals of gorillas and how they influence people's views of gorillas.

9. **D) is correct.** In this text, two brands of cream are being compared and contrasted.

10. **B) is correct.** Both passages indicate that habitats are diminishing, impacting access to food.

11. **A) is correct.** *Fortification* and *fortress* are synonyms. In the seventeenth century, the purpose of the fortress changed. This is a clue that *converted* means "a change in form or function."

12. **A) is correct.** The root *cred* means *believe*. The words *evidence, reviewed,* and *approved* are context clues hinting that something needs to be believed and accepted.

13. **D) is correct.** The author compares the food trucks to "a carnival of delicious treats," using the word *like*.

14. **B) is correct.** According to the passage, a baby achieves milestones in independent movement in this order. Use the ages and signal words to determine the order of events.

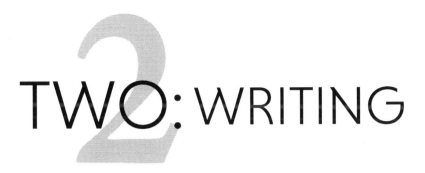

TWO: WRITING

Grammar

The English and Language Usage section will test your understanding of the basic rules of grammar. The first step in preparing for this section of the test is to review the parts of speech and the rules that accompany them. The good news is that you have been using these rules since you first began to speak. Even if you do not know a lot of the technical terms, many of these rules will be familiar to you. Some of the topics you might see include:

- matching pronouns with their antecedents
- matching verbs with their subjects
- ensuring that verbs are in the correct tense
- using correct capitalization
- distinguishing between types of sentences
- correcting sentence structure
- identifying parts of speech

NOUNS AND PRONOUNS

Nouns are people, places, or things. The subject of a sentence is typically a noun. For example, in the sentence "The hospital was very clean," the subject, *hospital*, is a noun; it is a place. **Pronouns** stand in for nouns and can be used to make sentences sound less repetitive. Take the sentence, "Sam stayed home from school because Sam was not feeling well." The word *Sam* appears twice in the same sentence. Instead, you can use the pronoun *he* to stand in for *Sam* and say, "Sam stayed home from school because he was not feeling well."

Because pronouns take the place of nouns, they need to agree both in number and gender with the noun they replace. So, a plural noun needs a plural pronoun, and a noun referring to something feminine needs a feminine pronoun. In the first sentence in this paragraph, for example, the plural pronoun *they* replaced the plural noun *pronouns*. There will usually be several questions on the English and Language Usage section that cover pronoun agreement, so it's good to get comfortable spotting pronouns.

HELPFUL HINT

SINGULAR PRONOUNS

- I, me, my, mine
- you, your, yours
- he, him, his
- she, her, hers
- it, its

PLURAL PRONOUNS

- we, us, our, ours
- they, them, their, theirs

Wrong: If a student forgets their homework, they will not receive a grade

Correct: If a student forgets his or her homework, he or she will not receive a grade.

Student is a singular noun, but *their* and *they* are plural pronouns. So, the first sentence is incorrect. To correct it, use the singular pronoun *his* or *her* or *he* or *she*.

Wrong: Everybody will receive their paychecks promptly.

Correct: Everybody will receive his or her paycheck promptly.

Everybody is a singular noun, but *their* is a plural pronoun. So, the first sentence is incorrect. To correct it, use the singular pronoun *his* or *her*.

Wrong: When nurses scrub in to surgery, you should wash your hands.

Correct: When nurses scrub in to surgery, they should wash their hands.

The first sentence begins in third-person perspective and then switches to second-person perspective. So, this sentence is incorrect. To correct it, use a third-person pronoun in the second clause.

Wrong: After the teacher spoke to the student, she realized her mistake.

Correct: After Mr. White spoke to his student, she realized her mistake. (*She* and *her* refer to the student.)

Correct: After speaking to the student, the teacher realized her own mistake. (*Her* refers to the teacher.)

The first sentence refers to a teacher and a student. But whom does *she* refer to, the teacher or the student? To eliminate the ambiguity, use specific names or state more specifically who made the mistake.

PRACTICE QUESTIONS

1. Which of the following lists includes all the nouns in the sentence?
   I have lived in Minnesota since August, but I still don't own a warm coat or gloves.
   A) coat, gloves
   B) I, coat, gloves
   C) Minnesota, August, coat, gloves
   D) I, Minnesota, August, warm, coat, gloves

2. In which of the following sentences do the nouns and pronouns not agree?
   A) After we walked inside, we took off our hats and shoes and hung them in the closet.
   B) The members of the band should leave her instruments in the rehearsal room.
   C) The janitor on duty should rinse out his or her mop before leaving for the day.
   D) When you see someone in trouble, you should always try to help them.

VERBS

A **verb** is the action of a sentence: it describes what the subject of the sentence is or is doing. Verbs must match the subject of the sentence in person and number, and must be in the proper tense—past, present, or future.

Person describes the relationship of the speaker to the subject of the sentence: first (I, we), second (you), and third (he, she, it, they). *Number* refers to whether the subject of the sentence is singular or plural. Verbs are conjugated to match the person and number of the subject.

HELPFUL HINT

Think of the subject and the verb as sharing a single s. If the subject ends with an s, the verb should not, and vice versa.

Table 2.1. Conjugating Verbs for Person

Person	Singular	Plural
First	I jump	we jump
Second	you jump	you jump
Third	he/she/it jumps	they jump

Wrong: The cat chase the ball while the dogs runs in the yard.

Correct: The cat chases the ball while the dogs run in the yard.

Cat is singular, so it takes a singular verb (which confusingly ends with an *s*); *dogs* is plural, so it needs a plural verb.

Wrong: The cars that had been recalled by the manufacturer was returned within a few months.

Correct: The cars that had been recalled by the manufacturer were returned within a few months.

Sometimes, the subject and verb are separated by clauses or phrases. Here, the subject *cars* is separated from the verb by the relatively long phrase "that had been recalled by the manufacturer," making it more difficult to determine how to correctly conjugate the verb.

Correct: The doctor and nurse work in the hospital.

Correct: Neither the nurse nor her boss was scheduled to take a vacation.

Correct: Either the patient or her parents need to sign the release forms.

When the subject contains two or more nouns connected by *and*, that subject becomes plural and requires a plural verb. Singular subjects joined by *or, either/or, neither/nor,* or *not only/but also* remain singular; when these words join plural and singular subjects, the verb should match the closest subject.

Finally, verbs must be conjugated for tense, which shows when the action happened. Some conjugations include helping verbs like *was, have, have been,* and *will have been.*

HELPFUL HINT

If the subject is separated from the verb, cross out the phrases between them to make conjugation easier.

Table 2.2. Verb Tenses

Tense	Past	Present	Future
Simple	I <u>gave</u> her a gift yesterday.	I <u>give</u> her a gift every day.	I <u>will give</u> her a gift on her birthday.
Continuous	I <u>was giving</u> her a gift when you got here.	I <u>am giving</u> her a gift; come in!	I <u>will be giving</u> her a gift at dinner.
Perfect	I <u>had given</u> her a gift before you got there.	I <u>have given</u> her a gift already.	I <u>will have given</u> her a gift by midnight.
Perfect continuous	Her friends <u>had been giving</u> her gifts all night when I arrived.	I <u>have been giving</u> her gifts every year for nine years.	I <u>will have been giving</u> her gifts on holidays for ten years next year.

Tense must also be consistent throughout the sentence and the passage. For example, the sentence *I was baking cookies and eat some dough* sounds strange. That is because the two verbs, *was baking* and *eat*, are in different tenses. *Was baking* occurred in the past; *eat*, on the other hand, occurs in the present. To make them consistent, change *eat* to *ate*.

Wrong: Because it will rain during the party last night, we had to move the tables inside.

Correct: Because it rained during the party last night, we had to move the tables inside.

All the verb tenses in a sentence need to agree both with each other and with the other information in the sentence. In the first sentence above, the tense does not match the other information in the sentence: *last night* indicates the past (*rained*), not the future (*will rain*).

PRACTICE QUESTIONS

3. Which of the following sentences contains an incorrectly conjugated verb?

    A) The brother and sister runs very fast.

    B) Neither Anne nor Suzy likes the soup.

    C) The mother and father love their new baby.

    D) Either Jack or Jill will pick up the pizza.

4. Which of the following sentences contains an incorrect verb tense?

    A) After the show ended, we drove to the restaurant for dinner.

    B) Anne went to the mall before she headed home.

    C) Johnny went to the movies after he cleans the kitchen.

    D) Before the alarm sounded, smoke filled the cafeteria.

ADJECTIVES AND ADVERBS

Adjectives provide more information about a noun in a sentence. Take the sentence, "The boy hit the ball." If you want your readers to know more about the noun *boy*, you could use an adjective to describe him: *the little boy, the young boy, the tall boy*.

Adverbs and adjectives are similar because they provide more information about a part of a sentence. However, adverbs do not describe nouns—that's an adjective's job. Instead, adverbs describe verbs, adjectives, and even other adverbs. For example, in the sentence "The doctor had recently hired a new employee," the adverb *recently* tells us more about how the action *hired* took place.

Adjectives, adverbs, and **modifying phrases** (groups of words that together modify another word) should be placed as close as possible to the word they modify. Separating words from their modifiers can create incorrect or confusing sentences.

> **Wrong:** Running through the hall, the bell rang and the student knew she was late.
>
> **Correct:** Running through the hall, the student heard the bell ring and knew she was late.

The phrase *running through the hall* should be placed next to *student*, the noun it modifies.

The suffixes *–er* and *–est* are often used to modify adjectives when a sentence is making a comparison. The suffix *–er* is used when comparing two things, and the suffix *–est* is used when comparing more than two.

> Anne is taller than Steve, but Steve is more coordinated.
>
> Of the five brothers, Billy is the funniest, and Alex is the most intelligent.

Adjectives longer than two syllables are compared using *more* (for two things) or *most* (for three or more things).

> **Wrong:** Of my two friends, Clara is the smartest.
>
> **Correct:** Of my two friends, Clara is smarter.

More and *most* should not be used in conjunction with *–er* and *–est* endings.

> **Wrong:** My most warmest sweater is made of wool.
>
> **Correct:** My warmest sweater is made of wool.

PRACTICE QUESTIONS

5. Which of the following lists includes all the adjectives in the sentence?
   The new chef carefully stirred the boiling soup and then lowered the heat.
   A) new, boiling
   B) new, carefully, boiling
   C) new, carefully, boiling, heat
   D) new, carefully, boiling, lowered, heat

6. Which of the following sentences contains an adjective error?

A) The new red car was faster than the old blue car.

B) Reggie's apartment is in the tallest building on the block.

C) The slice of cake was tastier than the brownie.

D) Of the four speeches, Jerry's was the most long.

OTHER PARTS OF SPEECH

Prepositions express the location of a noun or pronoun in relation to other words and phrases described in a sentence. For example, in the sentence "The nurse parked her car in a parking garage," the preposition *in* describes the position of the car in relation to the garage. Together, the preposition and the noun that follow it are called a **prepositional phrase**. In this example, the prepositional phrase is "in a parking garage."

Conjunctions connect words, phrases, and clauses. The conjunctions summarized in the acronym FANBOYS—For, And, Nor, But, Or, Yet, So—are called **coordinating conjunctions** and are used to join **independent clauses** (clauses that can stand alone as a complete sentence). For example, in the following sentence, the conjunction *and* joins together two independent clauses:

The nurse prepared the patient for surgery, <u>and</u> the doctor performed the surgery.

Other conjunctions, like *although*, *because*, and *if*, join together an independent and a **dependent clause** (which cannot stand on its own). Take the following sentence:

She had to ride the subway <u>because her car was broken</u>.

The clause *because her car was broken* cannot stand on its own.

Interjections, like *wow* and *hey*, express emotion and are most commonly used in conversation and casual writing.

PRACTICE QUESTIONS

Choose the word that best completes the sentence.

7. Her love _____ blueberry muffins kept her coming back to the bakery every week.

A) to

B) with

C) of

D) about

8. Christine left her house early on Monday morning, _____ she was still late for work.

A) but

B) and

C) for

D) or

Sentence Structure

PHRASES

To understand what a phrase is, you have to know about subjects and predicates. The **subject** is what the sentence is about; the **predicate** contains the verb and its modifiers.

The nurse at the front desk will answer any questions you have.

Subject: the nurse at the front desk

Predicate: will answer any questions you have

A **phrase** is a group of words that communicates only part of an idea because it lacks either a subject or a predicate. Phrases are categorized based on the main word in the phrase. A **prepositional phrase** begins with a preposition and ends with an object of the preposition, a **verb phrase** is composed of the main verb along with any helping verbs, and a **noun phrase** consists of a noun and its modifiers.

Prepositional phrase: The dog is hiding under the porch.

Verb phrase: The chef wanted to cook a different dish.

Noun phrase: The big red barn rests beside the vacant chicken house.

PRACTICE QUESTION

9. Identify the type of phrase underlined in the following sentence.

The new patient was assigned to the nurse with the most experience.

A) prepositional phrase

B) noun phrase

C) verb phrase

D) verbal phrase

CLAUSES

Clauses contain both a subject and a predicate. They can be either independent or dependent. An **independent** (or main) **clause** can stand alone as its own sentence.

The dog ate her homework.

Dependent (or subordinate) clauses cannot stand alone as their own sentences. They start with a subordinating conjunction, relative pronoun, or relative adjective, which will make them sound incomplete.

Because the dog ate her homework

A sentence can be classified as simple, compound, complex, or compound-complex based on the type and number of clauses it has.

Table 2.3. Sentences

Sentence type	Number of independent clauses	Number of dependent clauses
Simple	1	0
Compound	2 or more	0
Complex	1	1 or more
Compound-complex	2 or more	1 or more

HELPFUL HINT

On the test you will have to both identify and construct different kinds of sentences.

A **simple sentence** consists of one independent clause. Because there are no dependent clauses in a simple sentence, it can be a two-word sentence, with one word being the subject and the other word being the verb, such as *I ran*. However, a simple sentence can also contain prepositions, adjectives, and adverbs. Even though these additions can extend the length of a simple sentence, it is still considered a simple sentence as long as it does not contain any dependent clauses.

> San Francisco in the springtime is one of my favorite places to visit.

Although the sentence is lengthy, it is simple because it contains only one subject and one verb (*San Francisco* and *is*), modified by additional phrases.

Compound sentences have two or more independent clauses and no dependent clauses. Usually a comma and a coordinating conjunction (the FANBOYS: *For, And, Nor, But, Or, Yet,* and *So*) join the independent clauses, though semicolons can be used as well. The sentence "My computer broke, so I took it to be repaired" is compound.

> The game was canceled, but we will still practice on Saturday.

This sentence is made up of two independent clauses joined by a conjunction (*but*), so it is compound.

Complex sentences have one independent clause and at least one dependent clause. In the complex sentence "If you lie down with dogs, you'll wake up with fleas," the first clause is dependent (because of the subordinating conjunction *if*), and the second is independent.

> I love listening to the radio in the car because I can sing along as loud as I want.

> The sentence has one independent clause (*I love...car*) and one dependent (*because I...want*), so it is complex.

QUICK REVIEW

Can you write a simple, compound, complex, and compound-complex sentence using the same independent clause?

Compound-complex sentences have two or more independent clauses and at least one dependent clause. For example, the sentence *Even though David was a vegetarian, he went with his friends to steakhouses, but he focused on the conversation instead of the food,* is compound-complex.

I wanted to get a dog, but I have a fish because my roommate is allergic to pet dander.

This sentence has three clauses: two independent (*I wanted...dog* and *I have a fish*) and one dependent (*because my...dander*), so it is compound-complex.

PRACTICE QUESTIONS

10. Which of the following choices is a simple sentence?

A) Elsa drove while Erica navigated.

B) Betty ordered a fruit salad, and Sue ordered eggs.

C) Because she was late, Jenny ran down the hall.

D) John ate breakfast with his mother, brother, and father.

11. Which of the following sentences is a compound-complex sentence?

A) While they were at the game, Anne cheered for the home team, but Harvey rooted for the underdogs.

B) The rain flooded all of the driveway, some of the yard, and even part of the sidewalk across the street.

C) After everyone finished the test, Mr. Brown passed a bowl of candy around the classroom.

D) All the flowers in the front yard are in bloom, and the trees around the house are lush and green.

PUNCTUATION

The basic rules for using the major punctuation marks are given in the table below.

Table 2.4. How to Use Punctuation

Punctuation	Used for	Example
Period	ending sentences	Periods go at the end of complete sentences.
Question mark	ending questions	What's the best way to end a sentence?
Exclamation point	ending sentences that show extreme emotion	I'll never understand how to use commas!
Comma	joining two independent clauses (always with a coordinating conjunction)	Commas can be used to join clauses, but they must always be followed by a coordinating conjunction.
	setting apart introductory and nonessential words and phrases	Commas, when used properly, set apart extra information in a sentence.
	separating items in a list	My favorite punctuation marks include the colon, semicolon, and period.

Table 2.4. How to Use Punctuation (continued)

Punctuation	Used for	Example
Semicolon	joining together two independent clauses (never used with a conjunction)	I love exclamation points; they make sentences seem so exciting!
Colon	introducing a list, explanation, or definition	When I see a colon I know what to expect: more information.
Apostrophe	forming contractions	It's amazing how many people can't use apostrophes correctly.
	showing possession	Parentheses are my sister's favorite punctuation; she finds commas' rules confusing.
Quotation marks	indicating a direct quote	I said to her, "Tell me more about parentheses."

PRACTICE QUESTIONS

12. Which of the following sentences contains an error in punctuation?

    A) I love apple pie! John exclaimed with a smile.

    B) Jennifer loves Adam's new haircut.

    C) Billy went to the store; he bought bread, milk, and cheese.

    D) Alexandra hates raisins, but she loves chocolate chips.

13. Which punctuation mark correctly completes the sentence?

    *Sam, why don't you come with us for dinner_*

    A) .

    B) ?

    C) ;

    D) :

ANSWER KEY

1. **C) is correct.** *Minnesota* and *August* are proper nouns, and *coat* and *gloves* are common nouns. *I* is a pronoun, and *warm* is an adjective that modifies *coat*.

2. **B) is correct.** "The members of the band" is plural, so it should be replaced by the plural pronoun *their* instead of the singular *her*.

3. **A) is correct.** Choice A should read "The brother and sister run very fast." When the subject contains two or more nouns connected by *and*, the subject is plural and requires a plural verb.

4. **C) is correct.** Choice C should read "Johnny will go to the movies after he cleans the kitchen." It does not make sense to say that Johnny does something in the past (*went to the movies*) after doing something in the present (*after he cleans*).

5. **A) is correct.** *New* modifies the noun *chef*, and *boiling* modifies the noun *soup*. *Carefully* is an adverb modifying the verb *stirred*. *Lowered* is a verb, and *heat* is a noun.

6. **D) is correct.** Choice D should read, "Of the four speeches, Jerry's was the longest." The word *long* has only one syllable, so it should be modified with the suffix *–est*, not the word *most*.

7. **C) is correct.** The correct preposition is *of*.

8. **A) is correct.** In this sentence, the conjunction is joining together two contrasting ideas, so the correct answer is *but*.

9. **A) is correct.** The underlined section of the sentence is a prepositional phrase beginning with the preposition *with*.

10. **D) is correct.** Choice D contains one independent clause with one subject and one verb. Choices A and C are complex sentences because they each contain both a dependent and independent clause. Choice B contains two independent clauses joined by a conjunction and is therefore a compound sentence.

11. **A) is correct.** Choice A is a compound-complex sentence because it contains two independent clauses and one dependent clause. Despite its length, choice B is a simple sentence because it contains only one independent clause. Choice C is a complex sentence because it contains one dependent clause and one independent clause. Choice D is a compound sentence; it contains two independent clauses.

12. **A) is correct.** Choice A should use quotation marks to set off a direct quote: *"I love apple pie!" John exclaimed with a smile.*

13. **B) is correct.** The sentence is a question, so it should end with a question mark.

THREE: MATHEMATICS

Types of Numbers

Numbers are placed in categories based on their properties.

- A **natural number** is greater than zero and has no decimal or fraction attached. These are also sometimes called counting numbers. {1, 2, 3, 4, ...}

- **Whole numbers** are natural numbers and the number zero. {0, 1, 2, 3, 4, ...}

- **Integers** include positive and negative natural numbers and zero. {. . ., −4, −3, −2, −1, 0, 1, 2, 3, 4, ...}

- A **rational number** can be represented as a fraction. Any decimal part must terminate or resolve into a repeating pattern. Examples include −12, −$\frac{4}{5}$, 0.36, 7.$\overline{7}$, 26$\frac{1}{2}$, etc.

- An **irrational number** cannot be represented as a fraction. An irrational decimal number never ends and never resolves into a repeating pattern. Examples include −$\sqrt{7}$, π, and 0.34567989135 ...

- A **real number** is a number that can be represented by a point on a number line. Real numbers include all the rational and irrational numbers.

HELPFUL HINT

If a real number is a natural number (e.g. 50), then it is also an integer, a whole number, and a rational number.

Every natural number (except 1) is either a prime number or a composite number. A **prime number** is a natural number greater than 1 which can only be divided evenly by 1 and itself. For example, 7 is a prime number because it can only be divided by the numbers 1 and 7.

On the other hand, a **composite number** is a natural number greater than 1 which can be evenly divided by at least one other number besides 1 and itself. For example, 6 is a composite number because it can be divided by 1, 2, 3, and 6.

Composite numbers can be broken down into prime numbers using factor trees. For example, the number 54 is 2 × 27, and 27 is 3 × 9, and 9 is 3 × 3, as shown in Figure 3.1.

Once the number has been broken down into its simplest form, the composite number can be expressed as a product of prime factors. Repeated factors can be written using exponents. An **exponent** shows how many times a number should be multiplied by itself. As shown in the factor tree, the number 54 can be written as 2 × 3 × 3 × 3 or 2 × 3^3.

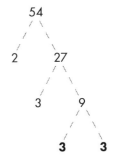

**Figure 3.1.
Factor Tree**

Scientific Notation

Scientific notation is a method of representing very large and small numbers in the form $a \times 10^n$ where a is a value between 1 and 10, and n is an integer. For example, the number 927,000,000 is written in scientific notation as 9.27×10^8. Multiplying 9.27 by 10 eight times gives 927,000,000. When performing operations with scientific notation, the final answer should be in the form $a \times 10^n$.

Table 3.1. Place Value

1,000,000	100,000	10,000	1,000	100	10	1	•	$\frac{1}{10}$	$\frac{1}{100}$
10^6	10^5	10^4	10^3	10^2	10^1	10^0		10^{-1}	10^{-2}
Millions	Hundred Thousands	Ten Thousands	Thousands	Hundreds	Tens	Ones	Decimal	Tenths	Hundreths

When adding and subtracting numbers in scientific notation, the power of 10 must be the same for all numbers. This results in like terms in which the a terms are added or subtracted and the 10^n remains unchanged. When multiplying numbers in scientific notation, multiply the a factors and add the exponents. For division, divide the a factors and subtract the exponents.

Positive and Negative Numbers

Positive numbers are greater than zero, and **negative numbers** are less than zero. Both positive and negative numbers can be shown on a **number line**.

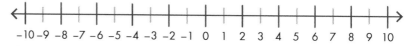

Figure 3.2. Number Line

Positive and negative numbers can be added, subtracted, multiplied, and divided. The sign of the resulting number is governed by a specific set of rules shown in the table below.

Table 3.2. Operations with Positive and Negative Numbers

Adding Real Numbers

Positve + Positive = Positive	$7 + 8 = 15$
Negative + Negative = Negative	$-7 + (-8) = -15$
Negative + Positive = Keep the sign of the number with the larger absolute value	$-7 + 8 = 1$ $7 + (-8) = -1$

Subtracting Real Numbers

Change the subtraction to addition, change the sign of the second number, and use addition rules.	
Negative − Positive = Negative	$-7 - 8 = -7 + (-8) = -15$
Positive − Negative = Positive	$7 - (-8) = 7 + 8 = 15$
Negative − Negative = Keep the sign of the number with the larger absolute value.	$-7 - (-8) = -7 + 8 = 1$ $-8 - (-7) = -8 + 7 = -1$
Positive − Positive = Positive if the first number is larger Negative if the second number is larger	$8 - 4 = 4$ $4 - 8 = -4$

Multiplying Real Numbers

Positive × Positive = Positive	$8 \times 4 = 32$
Negative × Negative = Positive	$-8 \times (-4) = 32$
Negative × Positive = Negative	$8 \times (-4) = -32$ $-8 \times 4 = -32$

Dividing Real Numbers

Positive ÷ Positive = Positive	$8 \div 4 = 2$
Negative ÷ Negative = Positive	$-8 \div (-4) = 2$
Positive ÷ Negative OR Negative ÷ Positive = Negative	$8 \div (-4) = -2$ $-8 \div 4 = -2$

PRACTICE QUESTIONS

Add or subtract the following real numbers:

6. $-18 + 12$

7. $-3.64 + (-2.18)$

8. $9.37 - 4.25$

9. $86 - (-20)$

Multiply or divide the following real numbers:

10. $\frac{10}{3}\left(-\frac{9}{5}\right)$

11. $\frac{-64}{-10}$

12. $(2.2)(3.3)$

13. $-52 \div 13$

Order of Operations

When solving a multi-step equation, the **order of operations** must be used to get the correct answer. Generally speaking, the problem should be worked in the following order: 1) parentheses and brackets; 2) exponents and square roots; 3) multiplication and division; 4) addition and subtraction. The acronym PEMDAS can be used to remember the order of operations.

Please Excuse (**My Dear**) (**Aunt Sally**)

1. **P** — Parentheses: Calculate expressions inside parentheses, brackets, braces, etc.

2. **E** — Exponents: Calculate exponents and square roots.

3. **M** — Multiply and **D** — Divide: Calculate any remaining multiplication and division in order from left to right.

4. **A** — Add and **S** — Subtract: Calculate any remaining addition and subtraction in order from left to right.

The steps "Multiply-Divide" and "Addition-Subtraction" go in order from left to right. In other words, divide before multiplying if the division problem is on the left.

For example, the expression $(3^2 - 2)^2 + (4)5^3$ is simplified using the following steps:

1. Parentheses: Because the parentheses in this problem contain two operations (exponents and subtraction), use the order of operations within the parentheses. Exponents come before subtraction. $(3^2 - 2)^2 + (4)5^3 = (9 - 2)^2 + (4)5^3 = (7)^2 + (4)5^3$

2. Exponents: $(7)^2 + (4)5^3 = 49 + (4)125$

3. Multiplication and division: $49 + (4)125 = 49 + 500$

4. Addition and subtraction: $49 + 500 = 549$

PRACTICE QUESTIONS

14. Simplify: $2(21 - 14) + 6 \div (-2) \times 3 - 10$

15. Simplify: $-3^2 + 4(5) + (5 - 6)^2 - 8$

16. Simplify: $\dfrac{(7 - 9)^3 + 8(10 - 12)}{4^2 - 5^2}$

Decimals and Fractions

DECIMALS

A **decimal** is a number that contains a decimal point. The place value for a decimal includes **tenths** (one place after the decimal point), **hundredths** (two places after the decimal point), **thousandths** (three places after the decimal point), etc.

5	4	•	3	2
5×10^1	4×10^0		3×10^{-1}	2×10^{-2}
5×10	4×1		$3 \times \frac{1}{10}$	$2 \times \frac{1}{100}$
50	4		0.3	0.02
Tens	Ones	Decimal Point	Tenths	Hundredths

$50 + 4 + 0.3 + 0.02 = 54.32$

Figure 3.3. Decimals and Place Value

Decimals can be added, subtracted, multiplied, and divided:

To add or subtract decimals, line up the decimal points and perform the operation, keeping the decimal point in the same place in the answer.

$$\begin{array}{r} 12.35 \\ + \ 3.63 \\ \hline = 15.98 \end{array}$$

To multiply decimals, first multiply the numbers without the decimal points. Then, add the number of decimal places to the right of the decimal point in the original numbers and place the decimal point in the answer so that there are that many places to the right of the decimal.

$$12.35 \times 3.63 =$$
$$1235 \times 363 = 448305 \rightarrow 44.8305$$

HELPFUL HINT

If you're unsure which way to move the decimal after multiplying, remember that changing the decimal should always make the final answer smaller.

When dividing decimals, move the decimal point to the right in order to make the divisor a whole number and move the decimal the same number of places in the dividend. Divide the numbers without regard to the decimal. Then, place the decimal point of the quotient directly above the decimal point of the dividend.

$$\frac{12.35}{3.63} = \frac{1235}{363} =$$

$$363 \overline{)1235.0} \quad 3.4$$

PRACTICE QUESTIONS

17. Simplify: $24.38 + 16.51 - 29.87$

FRACTIONS

A **fraction** is a number that can be written in the form $\frac{a}{b}$ where b is not equal to zero. The a part of the fraction is the numerator (top number) and b part of the fraction is the denominator (bottom number).

If the denominator of a fraction is greater than the numerator, the value of the fraction is less than 1 and it is called a **proper fraction** (e.g., $\frac{3}{5}$ is a proper fraction).

In an **improper fraction**, the denominator is less than the numerator and the value of the fraction is greater than one (e.g., $\frac{8}{3}$ is an improper fraction). An improper fraction can be written as a whole number or a mixed number. A **mixed number** has a whole number part and a proper fraction part. Improper fractions can be converted to mixed numbers by dividing the numerator by the denominator, which gives the whole number part, and the remainder becomes the numerator of the proper fraction part (for example: improper fraction $\frac{25}{9}$ is equal to mixed number $2\frac{7}{9}$ because 9 divides into 25 two times, with a remainder of 7).

Conversely, mixed numbers can be converted to improper fractions. To do so, determine the numerator of the improper fraction by multiplying the denominator by the whole number, then adding the numerator. The final number is written as the (now larger) numerator over the original denominator.

Fractions with the same denominator can be added or subtracted by simply adding or subtracting the numerators; the denominator will remain unchanged. If the fractions to be added or subtracted do not have a common denominator, the least common multiple of the denominators must be found. The quickest way to find a common denominator of a set of values is simply to multiply all the values together. The result might not be the least common denominator, but it will get the job done.

In the operation $\frac{2}{3} - \frac{1}{2}$, the common denominator will be a multiple of both 3 and 2. Multiples are found by multiplying the denominator by whole numbers until a common multiple is found:

- multiples of 3 are **3** (3 × 1), **6** (3 × 2), **9** (3 × 3) …
- multiples of 2 are **2** (2 × 1), **4** (2 × 2), **6** (2 × 3) …

Since 6 is the smallest multiple of both 3 and 2, it is the least common multiple and can be used as the common denominator. Both the numerator and denominator of each fraction should be multiplied by the appropriate whole number:

$$\frac{2}{3}\left(\frac{2}{2}\right) - \frac{1}{2}\left(\frac{3}{3}\right) = \frac{4}{6} - \frac{3}{6} = \frac{1}{6}.$$

When multiplying fractions, simply multiply each numerator together and each denominator together, reducing the result if possible. To divide two fractions, invert the second fraction (swap the numerator and denominator), then multiply normally. If there are any mixed numbers when multiplying or dividing, they should first be changed to improper fractions. Note that multiplying proper fractions creates a value smaller than either original value.

$$\frac{5}{6} \times \frac{2}{3} = \frac{10}{18} = \frac{5}{9}$$

$$\frac{5}{6} \div \frac{2}{3} = \frac{5}{6} \times \frac{3}{2} = \frac{15}{12} = \frac{5}{4}$$

PRACTICE QUESTIONS

20. Simplify: $2\frac{3}{5} + 3\frac{1}{4} - 1\frac{1}{2}$

21. Simplify: $\frac{7}{8}\left(3\frac{1}{3}\right)$

22. Simplify: $4\frac{1}{2} \div \frac{2}{3}$

CONVERTING BETWEEN FRACTIONS AND DECIMALS

A fraction is converted to a decimal by using long division until there is no remainder or a pattern of repeating numbers occurs.

$$\frac{1}{2} = 1 \div 2 = 0.5$$

To convert a decimal to a fraction, place the numbers to the right of the decimal over the appropriate base-10 power and simplify the fraction.

$$0.375 = \frac{375}{1000} = \frac{3}{8}$$

PRACTICE QUESTIONS

23. Write the fraction $\frac{7}{8}$ as a decimal.

24. Write the fraction $\frac{5}{11}$ as a decimal.

25. Write the decimal 0.125 as a fraction.

Rounding and Estimation

Rounding is a way of simplifying a complicated number. The result of rounding will be a less precise value that is easier to write or perform operations on. Rounding is performed to a specific place value, such as the thousands or tenths place.

The rules for rounding are as follows:

1. Underline the place value being rounded to.

2. Locate the digit one place value to the right of the underlined value. If this value is less than 5, keep the underlined value and replace all digits to the right of the underlined value with zero. If the value to the right of the underlined digit is more than 5, increase the underlined digit by one and replace all digits to the right of it with zero.

Estimation is when numbers are rounded and then an operation is performed. This process can be used when working with large numbers to find a close, but not exact, answer.

HELPFUL HINT

Estimation can often be used to eliminate answer choices on multiple choice tests without having to completely work the problem.

26. Round the number 138,472 to the nearest thousand.

27. The populations of five local towns are 12,341, 8,975, 9,431, 10,521, and 11,427. Estimate the population to the nearest 1,000 people.

Ratios

A **ratio** is a comparison of two numbers and can be represented as $\frac{a}{b}$ ($b \neq 0$), $a{:}b$, or a to b. The two numbers represent a constant relationship, not a specific value: for every a number of items in the first group, there will be b number of items in the second. For example, if the ratio of blue to red candies in a bag is 3:5, the bag will contain 3 blue candies for every 5 red candies. So the bag might contain 3 blue candies and 5 red candies, or it might contain 30 blue candies and 50 red candies, or 36 blue candies and 60 red candies. All of these values are representative of the ratio 3:5 (which is the ratio in its lowest, or simplest, terms).

To find the "whole" when working with ratios, simply add the values in the ratio. For example, if the ratio of boys to girls in a class is 2:3, the "whole" is five: 2 out of every 5 students are boys, and 3 out of every 5 students are girls.

28. There are 10 boys and 12 girls in a first grade class. What is the ratio of boys to the total number of students? What is the ratio of girls to boys?

29. A family spends $600 a month on rent, $400 on utilities, $750 on groceries, and $550 on miscellaneous expenses. What is the ratio of the family's rent to their total expenses?

Proportions

A **proportion** is an equation which states that two ratios are equal. Proportions are given in the form $\frac{a}{b} = \frac{c}{d}$, where the a and d terms are the extremes and the b and c terms are the means. A proportion is solved using **cross-multiplication** to create an equation with no fractional components: $\frac{a}{b} = \frac{c}{d} \rightarrow ad = bc$

30. Solve the proportion for x: $\frac{3 - 5x}{2} = \frac{-8}{3}$

31. A map is drawn such that 2.5 inches on the map equates to an actual distance of 40 miles. If the distance between two cities measured on the map is 17.25 inches, what is the actual distance between them in miles?

32. At a certain factory, every 4 out of 1,000 parts made will be defective. If in a month there are 125,000 parts made, how many of these parts will be defective?

Percentages

A **percent** (or percentage) means per hundred and is expressed with a percent symbol (%). For example, 54% means 54 out of every 100. A percent can be converted to a decimal by removing the % symbol and moving the decimal point two places to the left, while a decimal can be converted to a percent by moving the decimal point two places to the right and attaching the % sign.

A percent can be converted to a fraction by writing the percent as a fraction with 100 as the denominator and reducing. A fraction can be converted to a percent by performing the indicated division, multiplying the result by 100 and attaching the % sign.

The percent equation has three variables: the part, the whole, and the percent (which is expressed in the equation as a decimal). The equation, as shown below, can be rearranged to solve for any of these variables.

$$\text{part} = \text{whole} \times \text{percent}$$

$$\text{percent} = \frac{\text{part}}{\text{whole}}$$

$$\text{whole} = \frac{\text{part}}{\text{percent}}$$

This set of equations can be used to solve percent word problems. All that is needed is to identify the part, whole, and/or percent, then to plug those values into the appropriate equation and solve.

PRACTICE QUESTIONS

33. Write 18% as a fraction.

34. Write $\frac{3}{5}$ as a percent.

35. Write 1.125 as a percent.

36. Write 84% as a decimal.

37. In a school of 650 students, 54% of the students are boys. How many students are girls?

PERCENT CHANGE

Percent change problems involve a change from an original amount. Often percent change problems appear as word problems that include discounts, growth, or markups. In order to solve percent change problems, it is necessary to identify the percent change (as a decimal), the amount of change, and the original amount. (Keep in mind that one of these will be the value being solved for.) These values can then be plugged into the equations below:

$$\text{amount of change} = \text{original amount} \times \text{percent change}$$

$$\text{percent change} = \frac{\text{amount of change}}{\text{original amount}}$$

$$\text{original amount} = \frac{\text{amount of change}}{\text{percent change}}$$

Comparison of Rational Numbers

Rational numbers can be ordered from least to greatest (or greatest to least) by placing them in the order in which they fall on a number line. When comparing a set of fractions, it is often easiest to convert each value to a common denominator. Then, it is only necessary to compare the numerators of each fraction.

When working with numbers in multiple forms (for example, a group of fractions and decimals), convert the values so that the set contains only fractions or only decimals. When ordering negative numbers, remember that the negative number with the largest absolute value is furthest from 0 and is therefore the smallest number. (For example, -75 is smaller than -25.)

PRACTICE QUESTIONS

40. Order the following numbers from greatest to least: $-\frac{2}{3}, 1.2, 0, -2.1, \frac{5}{4}, -1, \frac{1}{8}$.

41. Order the following numbers from least to greatest: $\frac{1}{3}, -\frac{5}{6}, 1\frac{1}{8}, \frac{7}{12}, -\frac{3}{4}, -\frac{3}{2}$.

Algebraic Expressions

The foundation of algebra is the **variable**, an unknown number represented by a symbol (usually a letter such as x or a). Variables can be preceded by a **coefficient**, which is a constant (i.e., a real number) in front of the variable, such as $4x$ or $-2a$. An **algebraic expression** is any sum, difference, product, or quotient of variables and numbers (for example $3x^2$, $2x + 7y - 1$, and $\frac{5}{x}$ are algebraic expressions). **Terms** are any quantities that are added or subtracted (for example, the terms of the expression $x^2 - 3x + 5$ are x^2, $3x$, and 5). A **polynomial expression** is an algebraic expression where all the exponents on the variables are whole numbers. A polynomial with two terms is known as a **binomial**, and one with three terms is a **trinomial**.

PRACTICE QUESTION

42. If $m = 4$, find the value of the following expression: $5(m - 2)^3 + 3m^2 - \frac{m}{4} - 1$

Operations with Expressions
ADDING AND SUBTRACTING

Expressions can be added or subtracted by simply adding and subtracting **like terms**, which are terms with the same variable part (the variables must be the same, with the same exponents on each variable). For example, in the expressions $2x + 3xy - 2z$ and

$6y + 2xy$, the like terms are $3xy$ and $2xy$. Adding the two expressions yields the new expression $2x + 5xy - 2z + 6y$. Note that the other terms did not change; they cannot combine because they have different variables.

PRACTICE QUESTION

43. If $a = 12x + 7xy - 9y$ and $b = 8x - 9xz + 7z$, what is $a + b$?

DISTRIBUTING AND FACTORING

Often, simplifying expressions requires distributing and factoring, which can be seen as two sides of the same coin. **Distribution** multiplies each term in the first factor by each term in the second factor to clear off parentheses, while **factoring** reverses this process, taking a polynomial in standard form and writing it as a product of two or more factors.

When distributing a monomial through a polynomial, the expression outside the parentheses is multiplied by each term inside the parentheses. Remember, coefficients are multiplied and exponents are added, following the rules of exponents.

The first step in factoring a polynomial is always to "undistribute," or factor out, the greatest common factor (GCF) among the terms. The GCF is multiplied by, in parentheses, the expression that remains of each term when the GCF is divided out of each term. Factoring can be checked by multiplying the GCF factor through the parentheses again.

HELPFUL HINT

Operations with polynomials can always be checked by plugging the same value into both expressions.

PRACTICE QUESTIONS

44. Expand the following expression: $5x(x^2 - 2c + 10)$

45. Expand the following expression: $x(5 + z) - z(4x - z^2)$

Linear Equations

An **equation** states that two expressions are equal to each other. Polynomial equations are categorized by the highest power of the variables they contain. For instance, the highest power of any exponent of a linear equation is 1, a quadratic equation has a variable raised to the second power, a cubic equation has a variable raised to the third power, and so on.

SOLVING LINEAR EQUATIONS

Solving an equation means finding the value(s) of the variable that make the equation true. To solve a linear equation, it is necessary to manipulate the terms so that the variable being solved for appears alone on exactly one side of the equal sign while everything else in the equation is on the other side.

The way to solve linear equations is to "undo" all the operations that connect numbers to the variable of interest. Follow these steps:

1. Eliminate fractions by multiplying each side by the least common multiple of any denominators.

2. Distribute to eliminate parentheses, braces, and brackets.

3. Combine like terms.

HELPFUL HINT

On multiple-choice tests, you can avoid solving equations by just plugging the answer choices into the given equation to see which value makes the equation true.

4. Use addition or subtraction to collect all terms containing the variable of interest to one side, and all terms not containing the variable to the other side.

5. Use multiplication or division to remove coefficients from the variable being solved for.

Sometimes there are no numeric values in the equation, or there will be a mix of numerous variables and constants. The goal will be to solve the equation for one of the variables in terms of the other variables. In this case, the answer will be an expression involving numbers and letters instead of a numeric value.

PRACTICE QUESTIONS

46. Solve for x: $\left(\dfrac{100(x + 5)}{20} \right) = 1$.

47. Solve for x: $2(x + 2)^2 - 2x^2 + 10 = 20$

GRAPHS OF LINEAR EQUATIONS

The most common way to write a linear equation is **slope-intercept form**:

$$y = mx + b$$

In this equation, m is the **slope**, and b is the **y-intercept**. Slope is often described as "rise over run" because it is calculated as the difference in y-values (rise) over the difference in x-values (run). The slope of the line is also the **rate of change** of the dependent variable y with respect to the independent variable x. The y-intercept is the point where the line crosses the y-axis, or where x equals zero.

To graph a linear equation, identify the y-intercept and place that point on the y-axis. Then, starting at the y-intercept, use the slope to count up (or down if negative) the "rise" part of the slope and to the right the "run" part of the slope to find a second point. These points can then be connected to draw the line. To find the equation of a line, identify the y-intercept, if possible, on the graph and use two easily identifiable points to find the slope.

HELPFUL HINT

Use the phrase **begin, move** to remember that b is the y-intercept (where to begin) and m is the slope (how the line moves).

PRACTICE QUESTIONS

48. What is the equation of the following line?

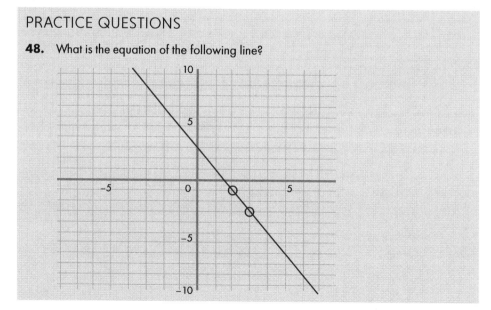

Building Equations

In word problems, it is often necessary to translate a verbal description of a relationship into a mathematical equation. No matter the problem, this process can be done using the same steps:

1. Read the problem carefully and identify what value needs to be solved for.

2. Identify the known and unknown quantities in the problem, and assign the unknown quantities a variable.

3. Create equations using the variables and known quantities.

4. Solve the equations.

5. Check the solution: Does it answer the question asked in the problem? Does it make sense?

HELPFUL HINT

Use the acronym **STAR** to remember word problem strategies. **S**earch the problem, **T**ranslate into an expression or equation, **A**nswer, and **R**eview.

PRACTICE QUESTIONS

50. A school is holding a raffle to raise money. There is a $3.00 entry fee, and each ticket costs $5.00. If a student paid $28.00, how many tickets did he buy?

51. Abby needs $395 to buy a new bicycle. She has borrowed $150 from her parents, and plans to earn the rest of the money working as a waitress. If she makes $10 per hour, how many hours will she need to work to pay for her new bicycle?

Inequalities

Inequalities are similar to equations, but both sides of the problem are not equal ($\neq$). Inequalities may be represented as follows: greater than ($>$), greater than or equal to ($\geq$), less than ($<$), or less than or equal to ($\leq$). For example, the statement "12 is less than 4 times x" would be written as $12 < 4x$.

Inequalities can be solved by manipulating them much like equations. However, the solution to an inequality is a set of numbers, not a single value. For example, simplifying $4x + 2 \leq 14$ gives the inequality $x \leq 3$, meaning every number less than 3 would also be included in the set of correct answers.

PRACTICE QUESTIONS

52. Solve the inequality: $4x + 10 > 58$

53. The students on the track team are buying new uniforms. T-shirts cost $12, pants cost $15, and a pair of shoes costs $45. If they have a budget of $2,500, write a mathematical sentence that represents how many of each item they can buy.

Units of Measurement

The standard units for the metric and American systems are shown below along with the prefixes used to express metric units.

Table 3.3. American and SI Units

Dimension	American	SI
Length	inch/foot/yard/mile	meter
Mass	ounce/pound/ton	gram
Volume	cup/pint/quart/gallon	liter
Force	pound-force	newton
Pressure	pound-force per square inch	pascal
Work and energy	cal/British thermal unit	joule
Temperature	Fahrenheit	kelvin
Charge	faraday	coulomb

Table 3.4. Metric Prefixes

Prefix	Symbol	Multiplication Factor
tera	T	1,000,000,000,000
giga	G	1,000,000,000
mega	M	1,000,000
kilo	k	1,000
hecto	h	100
deca	da	10
base unit	--	--
deci	d	0.1
centi	c	0.01
milli	m	0.001
micro	μ	0.000001
nano	n	0.000000001
pico	p	0.000000000001

Table 3.5. Conversion Factors

1 in. = 2.54 cm	1 lb. = 0.454 kg
1 yd. = 0.914 m	1 cal = 4.19 J
1 mi. = 1.61 km	$1°F = \frac{9}{5}°C + 32°C$
1 gal. = 3.785 L	$1\ cm^3 = 1\ mL$
1 oz. = 28.35 g	1 hr = 3600 s

HELPFUL HINT

A mnemonic device to help remember the metric system between kilo- and milli- is King Henry Drinks Under Dark Chocolate Moon (KHDUDCM).

Units can be converted within a single system or between systems. When converting from one unit to another unit, a **conversion factor** (a fraction used to convert a value with a unit into another unit) is used. For example, there are 2.54 centimeters in 1 inch, so the conversion factor from inches to centimeters is $\frac{2.54\ \text{centimeters}}{1\ \text{inch}}$.

To convert between units, multiply the original value by a conversion factor (or several if needed) so that the original units cancel, leaving the desired unit. Remember that the original value can be made into a fraction by placing it over 1.

$$\frac{3 \text{ inches}}{1} \times \frac{2.54 \text{ centimeters}}{1 \text{ inch}} = 7.62 \text{ centimeters}$$

Units can be canceled (meaning they disappear from the expression) when they appear on the top and the bottom of a fraction. If the same unit appears in the top (or bottom) of both fractions, you probably need to flip the conversion factor.

PRACTICE QUESTIONS

54. Convert 4.25 kilometers to meters.

55. Convert 12 feet to inches.

Geometric Figures
CLASSIFYING GEOMETRIC FIGURES

Geometric figures are shapes comprised of points, lines, or planes. A **point** is simply a location in space; it does not have any dimensional properties like length, area, or volume. A collection of points that extend infinitely in both directions is a **line**, and one that extends infinitely in only one direction is a **ray**. A section of a line with a beginning and end point is a **line segment**. Lines, rays, and line segments are examples of **one-dimensional** objects because they can only be measured in one dimension (length).

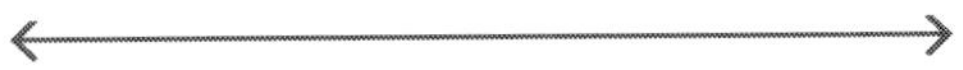

←————————————→

Figure 3.4. One-Dimensional Object

Lines, rays, and line segments can intersect to create **angles**, which are measured in degrees or radians. Angles between zero and 90 degrees are **acute**, and angles between 90 and 180 degrees are **obtuse**. An angle of exactly 90 degrees is a **right angle**, and two lines that form right angles are **perpendicular**. Lines that do not intersect are described as **parallel**.

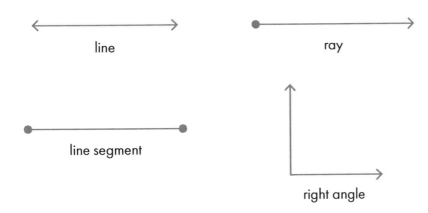

Figure 3.5A. Lines and Angles

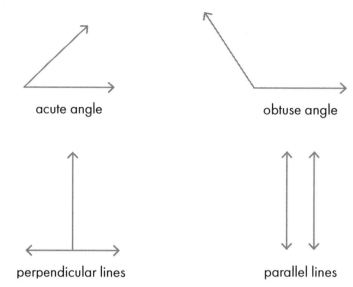

acute angle · obtuse angle

perpendicular lines · parallel lines

Figure 3.5B. Lines and Angles

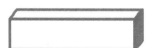

Figure 3.6. Two-Dimensional Object

Figure 3.7. Three-Dimensional Object

Two-dimensional objects can be measured in two dimensions—length and width. A **plane** is a two-dimensional object that extends infinitely in both directions. **Polygons** are two-dimensional shapes, such as triangles and squares, which have three or more straight sides. Regular polygons are polygons whose sides are all the same length.

Three-dimensional objects, such as cubes, can be measured in three dimensions—length, width, and height.

CALCULATING GEOMETRIC QUANTITIES

The **length**, or distance from one point to another on an object, can be determined using a tape measure or a ruler. The size of the surface of a two-dimensional object is its **area**. Generally, finding area involves multiplying one dimension of an object by another, such as length by width. For example, if a window is 3 feet long and 2 feet wide, its area would be 6 ft^2.

The distance around a two-dimensional figure is its **perimeter**, which can be found by adding the lengths of all the sides. The distance around a circle is referred to as its **circumference**.

Table 3.6. Area and Perimeter of Basic Shapes

Shape	Example	Area	Perimeter
Triangle		$A = \frac{1}{2} bh$	$P = s_1 + s_2 + s_3$
Square		$A = s^2$	$P = 4s$

Shape	Example	Area	Perimeter
Rectangle		$A = l \times w$	$P = 2l + 2w$
Trapezoid		$A = \frac{1}{2} h(b_1 + b_2)$	$P = b_1 + b_2 + l_1 + l_2$
Circle		$A = \pi r^2$	$C = 2\pi r$
Sector		$A = \frac{x°}{360°}(\pi r^2)$	arc length $= \frac{x°}{360°}(2\pi r)$

For the rectangle below, the area would be 8 m² because 2 m × 4 m = 8 m². The perimeter of the rectangle would be $P = 2l + 2w = 2(4 \text{ m}) + 2(2 \text{ m}) = 12$ m.

The **surface area** of a three-dimensional object can be figured by adding the areas of all the sides. For example, the box below is 4 feet long, 3 feet wide, and 1 foot deep. The surface area is found by adding the areas of each face:

- top: 4 ft × 3 ft = 12 ft²
- bottom: 4 ft × 3 ft = 12 ft²
- front: 4 ft × 1 ft = 4 ft²
- back: 4 ft × 1 ft = 4 ft²
- right: 1 ft × 3 ft = 3 ft²
- left: 1 ft × 3 ft = 3 ft²

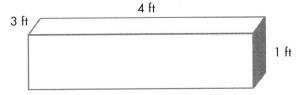

Figure 3.8. Surface Area

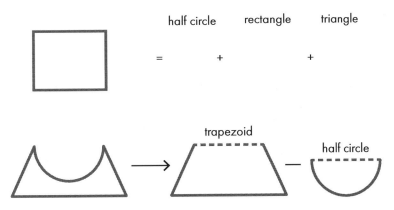

Figure 3.9. Compound Shapes

The KNAT may also ask test takers to find the perimeter and area of compound shapes, which will include parts of circles, squares, triangles, or other polygons joined together to create an irregular shape. For these types of problems, the first step is to divide the figure into shapes whose area (or perimeter) can easily be solved for. Then, solve each part separately and add (or subtract) the parts together for the final answer.

PRACTICE QUESTIONS

56. What is the area of the figure shown below?

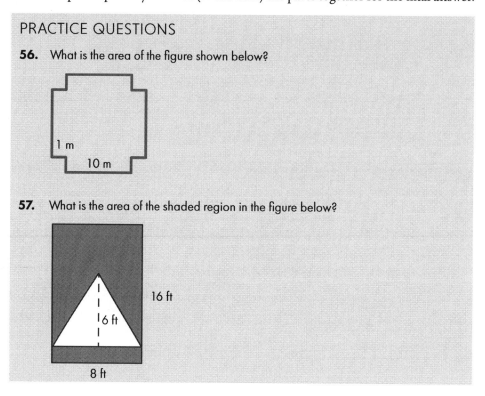

57. What is the area of the shaded region in the figure below?

Statistics

Statistics is the study of data. Analyzing data requires using **measures of central tendency** (mean, median, and mode) to identify trends or patterns.

The **mean** is the average; it is determined by adding all outcomes and then dividing by the total number of outcomes. For example, the average of the data set {16, 19, 19, 25, 27, 29, 75} is equal to $\frac{16 + 19 + 19 + 25 + 27 + 29 + 75}{7} = \frac{210}{7} = 30$.

The **median** is the number in the middle when the data set is arranged in order from least to greatest. For example, in the data set {16, 19, 19, **25**, 27, 29, 75}, the median is 25. When a data set contains an even number of values, finding the median requires averaging the two middle values. In the data set {75, 80, 82, 100}, the two numbers in the middle are 80 and 82. Consequently, the median will be the average of these two values: $\frac{80 + 82}{2} = 81$.

Finally, the **mode** is the most frequent outcome in a data set. In the set {16, 19, 19, 25, 27, 29, 75}, the mode is 19 because it occurs twice, which is more than any of the other numbers. If several values appear an equal, and most frequent, number of times, both values are considered the mode. If every value in a data set appears only once, the data set has no mode.

HELPFUL HINT

Mode is <u>most</u> common. Median is in the middle (like a median in the road). Mean is average.

Other useful indicators include range and outliers. The **range** is the difference between the highest and the lowest values in a data set. For example, the range of the set {16, 19, 19, 25, 27, 29, 75} is 75 − 16 = 59.

Outliers, or data points that are much different from other data points, should be noted as they can skew the central tendency. In the data set {16, 19, 19, 25, 27, 29, 75}, the value 75 is far outside the other values and raises the value of the mean. Without the outlier, the mean is much closer to the other data points.

- $\dfrac{16 + 19 + 19 + 25 + 27 + 29 + 75}{7} = \dfrac{210}{7} = 30$
- $\dfrac{16 + 19 + 19 + 25 + 27 + 29}{6} = \dfrac{135}{6} = 22.5$

Generally, the median is a better indicator of a central tendency if outliers are present to skew the mean.

Trends in a data set can also be seen by graphing the data as a dot plot. The distribution of the data can then be described based on the shape of the graph. A **symmetric** distribution looks like two mirrored halves, while a **skewed** distribution is weighted more heavily toward the right or the left. Note the direction of the skew describes the side of the graph with fewer data points. In a **uniform** data set, the points are distributed evenly along the graph.

A symmetric or skewed distribution may have peaks, or sets of data points that appear more frequently. A **unimodal** distribution has one peak while a **bimodal** distribution has two peaks. A normal (or bell-shaped) distribution is a special symmetric, unimodal graph with a specific distribution of data points.

PRACTICE QUESTIONS

58. Which of the following best describes the distribution of the graph?

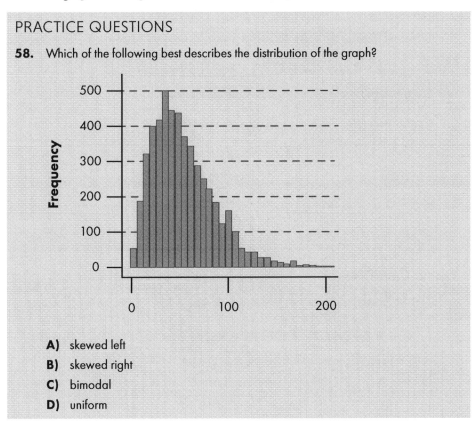

A) skewed left

B) skewed right

C) bimodal

D) uniform

Data Presentation

Data can be presented in a variety of ways. In addition to a simple table, there are a number of different graphs and charts that can be used to visually represent data. The most appropriate type of graph or chart depends on the data being displayed.

Box plots (also called box and whisker plots) show data using the median, range, and outliers of a data set. They provide a helpful visual guide, showing how data is distributed around the median. In the example below, 70 is the median and the range is 0 – 100, or 100.

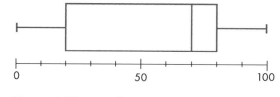

Figure 3.10. Box Plot

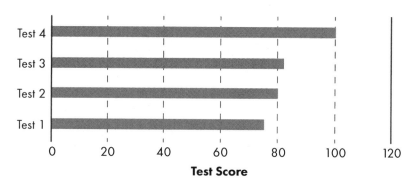

Figure 3.11. Bar Graph

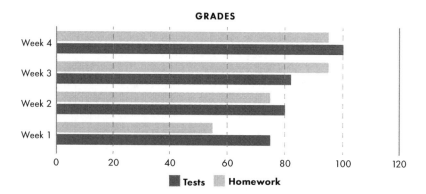

Figure 3.12. Double Bar Graph

Bar graphs use bars of different lengths to compare data. The independent variable on a bar graph is grouped into categories such as months, flavors, or locations, and the dependent variable is a quantity. Thus, comparing the length of bars provides a visual guide to the relative amounts in each category. **Double bar graphs** show more than one data set on the same set of axes.

Histograms similarly use bars to compare data, but the independent variable is a continuous variable that has been "binned" or divided into categories. For example, the time of day can be broken down into 8:00 a.m. to 12:00 p.m., 12:00 p.m. to 4:00 p.m., and so on. Usually (but not always), a gap is included between the bars of a bar graph but not a histogram. The bars of a bar graph show actual data, but the bars (or bins) of a histogram show the frequency of the data in various ranges.

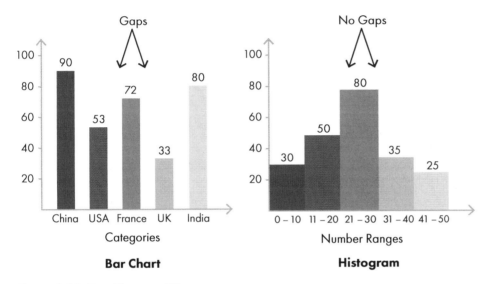

Figure 3.13. Bar Chart vs. Histogram

Dot plots display the frequency of a value or event data graphically using dots, and thus can be used to observe the distribution of a data set. Typically, a value or category is listed on the *x*-axis, and the number of times that value appears in the data set is represented by a line of vertical dots. Dot plots make it easy to see which values occur most often.

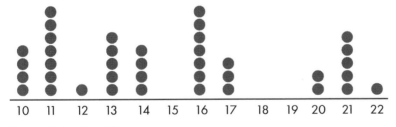

Figure 3.14. Dot Plot

Scatter plots use points to show relationships between two variables which can be plotted as coordinate points. One variable describes a position on the *x*-axis, and the other a point on the *y*-axis. Scatter plots can suggest relationships between variables. For example, both variables might increase together, or one may increase when the other decreases.

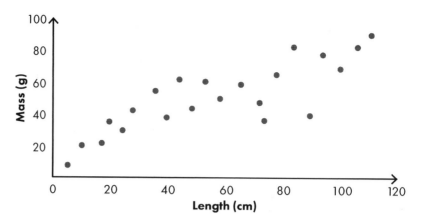

Figure 3.15. Scatter Plot

Line graphs show changes in data by connecting points on a scatter graph using a line. These graphs will often measure time on the *x*-axis and are used to show trends in the data, such as temperature changes over a day or school attendance throughout the year. **Double line graphs** present two sets of data on the same set of axes.

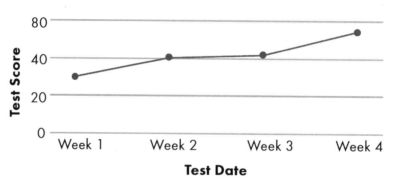

Figure 3.16. Line Graph

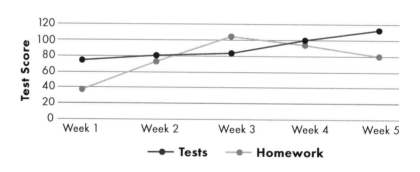

Figure 3.17. Double Line Graph

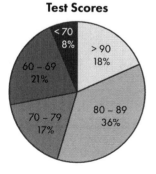

Figure 3.18. Circle Graph

Circle graphs (also called pie charts) are used to show parts of a whole: the "pie" is the whole, and each "slice" represents a percentage or part of the whole.

PRACTICE QUESTION

60. Students are asked if they prefer vanilla, chocolate, or strawberry ice cream. The results are tallied on the following table.

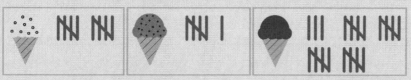

Four students display the information from the table in a bar graph. Which student completes the bar graph correctly?

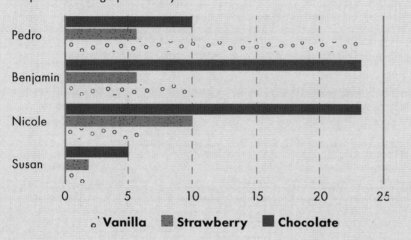

A) Pedro

B) Benjamin

C) Nicole

D) Susan

1. **Natural**, **whole**, **integer**, and **rational** (72 can be written as the fraction $\frac{72}{1}$).

2. **Rational** (The number is a fraction.)

3. **Irrational** (The number cannot be written as a fraction, and written as a decimal it is approximately 2.2360679... Notice this decimal does not terminate, nor does it have a repeating pattern.)

4. In order to add, the exponents of 10 must be the same. Change the first number so the power of 10 is 2:
   $3.8 \times 10^3 = 3.8 \times 10 \times 10^2 = 38 \times 10^2$
   Add the terms together and write the number in proper scientific notation:
   $38 \times 10^2 + 4.7 \times 10^2 = 42.7 \times 10^2 = \mathbf{4.27 \times 10^3}$

5. Multiply the factors and add the exponents on the base of 10:
   $(8.1 \times 1.4)(10^{-5} \times 10^7) = 11.34 \times 10^2$
   Write the number in proper scientific notation: (Place the decimal so that the first number is between 1 and 10 and adjust the exponent accordingly.)
   $11.34 \times 10^2 = \mathbf{1.134 \times 10^3}$

6. Since $|-18| > |12|$, the answer is negative. $|-18| - |12| = 6$. So the answer is **−6**.

7. Adding two negative numbers results in a negative number. Add the values: **−5.82**

8. **5.12**

9. Change the subtraction to addition, change the sign of the second number, then add:
   $86 - (-20) = 86 + (+20) = \mathbf{106}$

10. Multiply the numerators, multiply the denominators, then simplify: $-\frac{90}{15} = \mathbf{-6}$

11. A negative divided by a negative is a positive number: **6.4**

12. The parentheses indicate multiplication: **7.26**

13. A negative divided by a positive is negative: **−4**

14. Calculate the expressions inside the parenthesis:
    $2(21 - 14) + 6 \div (-2) \times 3 - 10 =$
    $2(7) + 6 \div (-2) \times 3 - 10$
    There are no exponents or radicals, so perform multiplication and division from left to right:
    $2(7) + 6 \div (-2) \times 3 - 10 =$
    $14 + 6 \div (-2) \times 3 - 10 =$
    $14 + (-3) \times 3 - 10 =$
    $14 + (-9) - 10$
    Lastly, perform addition and subtraction from left to right:
    $14 + (-9) - 10 = 5 - 10 = \mathbf{-5}$

15. Calculate the expressions inside the parentheses:

$-(3)^2 + 4(5) + (5 - 6)^2 - 8 =$

$-(3)^2 + 4(5) + (-1)^2 - 8$

Simplify exponents and radicals:

$-(3)^2 + 4(5) + (-1)^2 - 8 =$

$-9 + 4(5) + 1 - 8$

Note that $-(3)^2 = -1(3)^2 = -9$ but $(-1)^2 = (-1)(-1) = 1$

Perform multiplication and division from left to right:

$-9 + 4(5) + 1 - 8 =$

$-9 + 20 + 1 - 8$

Lastly, perform addition and subtraction from left to right:

$-9 + 20 + 1 - 8 =$

$11 + 1 - 8 = 12 - 8 =$ **4**

16. Simplify the top and bottom expressions separately using the same steps described above:

$$\frac{(-2)^3 + 8(-2)}{4^2 - 5^2} = \frac{-8 + (-16)}{16 - 25} = \frac{-24}{-9} = \frac{8}{3}$$

17. Apply the order of operations left to right:

$24.38 + 16.51 = 40.89$

$40.89 - 29.87 =$ **11.02**

18. Multiply the numbers ignoring the decimals: $104 \times 182 = 18{,}928$

The original problem includes two decimal places (10.4 has one place after the decimal point and 18.2 has one place after the decimal point), so place the decimal point in the answer so that there are two places after the decimal point. Estimating is a good way to check the answer ($10.4 \approx 10$, $18.2 \approx 18$, $10 \times 18 = 180$)

$18{,}928 \rightarrow$ **189.28**

19. The divisor is 2.5. Move the decimal one place to the right (multiply 2.5 by 10) so that the divisor is a whole number. Since the decimal point of the divisor was moved one place to the right, the decimal point in the dividend must be moved one place to the right (multiplying it by 10 as well).

$80 \rightarrow 800$ and $2.5 \rightarrow 25$

Divide normally: $800 \div 25 =$ **32**

20. The first step is to change each fraction so it has a denominator of 20, which is the LCD of 5, 4, and 2:

$2\frac{3}{5} + 3\frac{1}{4} - 1\frac{1}{2} = 2\frac{12}{20} + 3\frac{5}{20} - 1\frac{10}{20}$

Next, add and subtract the whole numbers together and the fractions together:

$2 + 3 - 1 = 4$

$\frac{12}{20} + \frac{5}{20} - \frac{10}{20} = \frac{7}{20}$

Lastly, combine to get the final answer (a mixed number): $\mathbf{4\frac{7}{20}}$

21. Change the mixed number to an improper fraction: $3\frac{1}{3} = \frac{10}{3}$

Multiply the numerators together and the denominators together, and then reduce the fraction:

$$\frac{7}{8}\left(\frac{10}{3}\right) = \frac{7 \times 10}{8 \times 3} = \frac{70}{24} = \frac{35}{12} = 2\frac{11}{12}$$

22. Change the mixed number to an improper fraction. Then, multiply the first fraction by the reciprocal of the second fraction and simplify:

$$\frac{9}{2} \div \frac{2}{3} = \frac{9}{2} \times \frac{3}{2} = \frac{27}{4} = 6\frac{3}{4}$$

23. Divide the denominator into the numerator using long division:

```
        0.875
    8 | 7.0000
        -64
         60
        -56
         60
        -56
         40
        -40
          0
```

24. Dividing using long division yields a repeating decimal:

```
         0.4545
    11 | 5.0000
         -44
          60
         -55
          50
         -44
          60
         -55
           5
```

25. Place the numbers to the right of the decimal (125) in the numerator. There are three numbers, so put the number 1000 in the denominator, and then reduce: $\frac{125}{1000} = \frac{1}{8}$

26. The 8 is in the thousands place, and the number to its right is a 4. Because 4 is less than 5, the 8 remains and all numbers to the right become zero:

$138,472 \approx \mathbf{138,000}$

27. Round each value to the thousands place and add:

$12,341 \approx 12,000$

$8,975 \approx 9,000$

$9,431 \approx 9,000$

$10,521 \approx 11,000$

$11,427 \approx 11,000$

$12,000 + 9,000 + 9,000 + 11,000 + 11,000 = \mathbf{52,000}$

28. There are 22 total students in the class. The ratio can be written as $\frac{10}{22}$, and reduced to $\frac{5}{11}$. The ratio of girls to boys is **12:10 or 6:5**.

29. The family's total expenses for the month add up to $2,300. The ratio of the rent to total amount of expenses can be written as $\frac{600}{2300}$ and reduced to $\frac{6}{23}$.

30. Start by cross multiplying:
$\frac{3-5}{2} = \frac{-8}{3} \rightarrow 3(3 - 5x) = 2(-8)$
Then, solve the equation:
$9 - 15x = -16$
$-15x = -25$
$x = \frac{-25}{-15} = \frac{5}{3}$

31. Write a proportion where x equals the actual distance and each ratio is written as inches:miles.
$\frac{2.5}{40} = \frac{17.25}{x}$
Then, cross-multiply and divide to solve: $2.5x = 690$
$x = 276$
The two cities are 276 miles apart.

32. Write a proportion in which x is the number of defective parts made and both ratios are written as defective parts:total parts.
$\frac{4}{1000} = \frac{x}{125,000}$
Then, cross-multiply and divide to solve for x: $1000x = 500,000$
$x = 500$
There are 500 defective parts for the month.

33. The percent is written as a fraction over 100 and reduced: $\frac{18}{100} = \frac{9}{50}$

34. Dividing 5 by 3 gives the value 0.6, which is then multiplied by 100: **60%**.

35. The decimal point is moved two places to the right: **112.5%**.

36. The decimal point is moved two places to the left: 84% = **0.84**.

37. The first step is to find the percent of students who are girls by subtracting from 100%:
100% − 54% = 46%
Next, identify the variables and plug into the appropriate equation:
percent = 46% = 0.46
whole = 650 students
part = ?
part = whole × percent = 0.46 × 650 = 299
There are 299 girls.

38. The first step is to identify the necessary values. These can then be plugged into the appropriate equation:
original amount = 1,500
percent change = 45% = 0.45
amount of change = ?
amount of change = original amount × percent change = 1,500 × 0.45 = 675

To find the new price, subtract the amount of change from the original price:

1,500 − 675 = 825 → The final price is **$825**.

39. Identify the necessary values and plug into the appropriate equation:

original amount = 100,000

amount of change = 120,000 − 100,000 = 20,000

percent change = ?

percent change = $\frac{\text{amount of change}}{\text{original amount}}$

= $\frac{20,000}{100,000}$ = 0.20

To find the percent growth, multiply by 100: 0.20 × 100 = **20%**

40. Change each fraction to a decimal:

$-\frac{2}{3} = -0.\overline{66}$

$\frac{5}{4} = 1.25$

$\frac{1}{8} = 0.125$

Now place the decimals in order from greatest to least:

1.25, 1.2, 0.125, 0, −0.$\overline{66}$, −1, −2.1

Lastly, convert back to fractions if the problem requires it:

$\frac{5}{4}$, **1.2,** $\frac{1}{8}$, **0,** $-\frac{2}{3}$, **−1, −2.1**

41. Convert each value using the least common denominator value of 24:

$\frac{1}{3} = \frac{8}{24}$

$-\frac{5}{6} = -\frac{20}{24}$

$1\frac{1}{8} = \frac{9}{8} = \frac{27}{24}$

$\frac{7}{12} = \frac{14}{24}$

$-\frac{3}{4} = -\frac{18}{24}$

$-\frac{3}{2} = -\frac{36}{24}$

Next, put the fractions in order from least to greatest by comparing the numerators:

$-\frac{36}{24}, -\frac{20}{24}, -\frac{18}{24}, \frac{8}{24}, \frac{14}{24}, \frac{27}{24}$

Finally, put the fractions back in their original form if the problem requires it:

$-\frac{3}{2}$, $-\frac{5}{6}$, $-\frac{3}{4}$, $\frac{1}{3}$, $\frac{7}{12}$, $1\frac{1}{8}$

42. First, plug the value 4 in for m in the expression:

$5(m − 2)^3 + 3m^2 − \frac{m}{4} − 1$

$= 5(4 − 2)^3 + 3(4)^2 − \frac{4}{4} − 1$

Then, simplify using PEMDAS:

P: $5(2)^3 + 3(4)^2 − \frac{4}{4} − 1$

E: $5(8) + 3(16) − \frac{4}{4} − 1$

M and D, working left to right: 40 + 48 − 1 − 1

A and S, working left to right: **86**

43. The only like terms in both expressions are $12x$ and $8x$, so these two terms will be added, and all other terms will remain the same:

$a + b = (12x + 8x) + 7xy - 9y - 9xz + 7z$

$= \mathbf{20x + 7xy - 9y - 9xz + 7z}$

44. The term outside the parentheses must be distributed and multiplied by all three terms inside the parentheses:

$(5x)(x^2) = 5x^3$

$(5x)(-2c) = -10xc$

$(5x)(10) = 50x$

$5x(x^2 - 2c + 10) \rightarrow \mathbf{5x^3 - 10xc + 50x}$

45. Start by distributing for each set of parentheses:

$x(5 + z) - z(4x - z^2)$

Notice that $-z$ is distributed and that $(-z)(-z^2) = +z^3$. Failing to distribute the negative is a very common error.

$5x + xz - 4zx + z^3$

Note that xz is a like term with zx (commutative property), and they can therefore be combined.

Now combine like terms and place terms in the appropriate order (highest exponents first): $\mathbf{z^3 - 3xz + 5x}$

46. To cancel out the denominator, multiply both sides by 20:

$20\dfrac{100(x + 5)}{20} = 1 \times 20$

$100(x + 5) = 20$

Next, distribute 100 through the parentheses:

$100(x + 5) = 20$

$100x + 500 = 20$

"Undo" the +500 by subtracting 500 from both sides of the equation to isolate the variable term: $100x = -480$

Finally, "undo" the multiplication by 100: divide by 100 on both sides to solve for x:

$\mathbf{x = \dfrac{-480}{100} = -4.8}$

47. First, simplify the left-hand side of the equation using order of operations and combining like terms.

$2(x + 2)^2 - 2x^2 + 10 = 20$

Do the exponent first: $2(x + 2)(x + 2) - 2x^2 + 10 = 20$

FOIL: $2(x^2 + 4x + 4) - 2x^2 + 10 = 20$

Distribute the 2: $2x^2 + 8x + 8 - 2x^2 + 10 = 20$

Combine like terms on the left-hand side: $8x + 18 = 20$

Now, isolate the variable.

"Undo" +18 by subtracting 18 from both sides: $8x + 18 = 20$

$8x = 2$

"Undo" multiplication by 8 by dividing both sides by 8: $\mathbf{x = \dfrac{2}{8}}$ **or** $\mathbf{\dfrac{1}{4}}$

48. The y-intercept can be identified on the graph as (0, 3). Thus, $b = 3$.

To find the slope, choose any two points and plug the values into the slope equation. The two points chosen here are $(2, -1)$ and $(3, -3)$.

$$m = \frac{(-3) - (-1)}{3 - 2} = \frac{-2}{1} = -2$$

Replace m with -2 and b with 3 in $y = mx + b$.

The equation of the line is **$y = -2x + 3$**.

49. Rearrange the equation into slope-intercept form by solving the equation for y. Isolate $-2y$ by subtracting $6x$ and adding 8 to both sides of the equation.

$-2y = -6x + 8$

Divide both sides by -2:

$$y = \frac{-6x + 8}{-2}$$

Simplify the fraction.

$y = 3x - 4$

The slope is 3, since it is the coefficient of x.

50. The problem is asking for the number of tickets. First, identify the quantities:

number of tickets = x

cost per ticket = 5

cost for x tickets = $5x$

total cost = 28

entry fee = 3

Now, set up an equation. The total cost for x tickets will be equal to the cost for x tickets plus the $3 entry fee: $5x + 3 = 28$

Now solve the equation:

$5x + 3 = 28$

$5x = 25$

$x = 5$

The student bought 5 tickets.

51. The problem asks for the number of hours Abby will have to work. First, identify the quantities:

number of hours = x

amount earned per hour = 10

amount of money earned = $10x$

price of bicycle = 395

money borrowed = 150

Now, set up an equation. The amount of money she has borrowed plus the money she earned as a waitress needs to equal the cost of the bicycle: $10x + 150 = 395$

Now solve the equation:

$10x + 150 = 395$

$10x = 245$

$x = 24.5$ hours

She will need to work 24.5 hours.

52. Inequalities can be solved using the same steps used to solve equations. Start by subtracting 10 from both sides:

$4x + 10 > 58$

$4x > 48$

Now divide by 4 to isolate x: **$x > 12$**

53. They have to spend less than \$2,500 on uniforms, so this problem is an inequality. First, identify the quantities:

number of t-shirts = t

total cost of t-shirts = $12t$

number of pants = p

total cost of pants = $15p$

number of pairs of shoes = s

total cost of shoes = $45s$

The cost of all the items must be less than \$2,500: **$12t + 15p + 45s < 2{,}500$**

54. $4.25 \text{ km} \left(\frac{1000 \text{ m}}{1 \text{ km}} \right) = \textbf{4250 m}$

55. $12 \text{ ft} \left(\frac{12 \text{ in}}{1 \text{ ft}} \right) = \textbf{144 in}$

56. The figure can be broken apart into three rectangles:

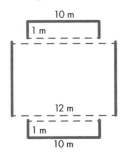

The area of each smaller rectangle is 1 m × 10 m = 10 m². The area of the larger rectangle is 10 m × 12 m = 120 m². Together, the area of the three shapes is 10 m² + 10 m² + 120 m² = **140 m²**

57. The area of the shaded region is the area of the rectangle minus the area of the triangle:

rectangle – triangle = (8 ft × 16 ft) – (0.5 × 8 ft × 6 ft) = 128 ft² – 24 ft² = **104 ft²**

58. **B) is correct.** The graph is skewed right because there are fewer data points on the right half.

59. **C) is correct.** The mean is the average: $\frac{14 + 18 + 11 + 28 + 23 + 14}{6} = \frac{108}{6} = \textbf{18}$

60. **B) is correct.** Benjamin's bar graph indicates that ten students prefer vanilla, six students prefer strawberry, and twenty-three students prefer chocolate ice cream.

FOUR: SCIENCE

Anatomical Terminology

THE BIOLOGICAL HIERARCHY

Organisms are living things consisting of at least one cell, which is the smallest unit of life that can reproduce on its own. Unicellular organisms, such as the amoeba, are made up of only one cell, while multicellular organisms are comprised of many cells. In a multicellular organism, the cells are grouped together into **tissues**, and these tissues are grouped into **organs**, which perform a specific function. The heart, for example, is the organ that pumps blood throughout the body. Organs are further grouped into **organ systems**, such as the digestive or respiratory systems.

A system is a collection of interconnected parts that make up a complex whole with defined boundaries. Systems may be closed, meaning nothing passes in or out of them, or open, meaning they have inputs and outputs. Organ systems are open and will have a number of inputs and outputs.

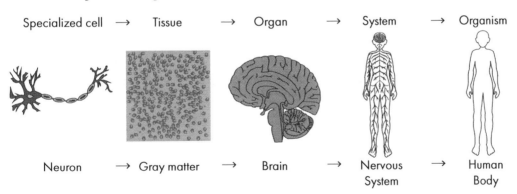

Specialized cell → Tissue → Organ → System → Organism

Neuron → Gray matter → Brain → Nervous System → Human Body

Figure 4.1. The Biological Hierarchy

DIRECTIONAL TERMS

Learning anatomy requires an understanding of the terminology used to describe the location of a particular structure. Anatomical science uses common terms to describe spatial relationships, often in pairs of opposites. These terms usually refer to the position of a structure in an organism that is upright with respect to its environment (e.g., in its typical orientation while moving forward).

Table 4.1. Directional Terms

Term	Meaning	Example
inferior	away from the head	The pelvis is inferior to the head.
superior	closer to the head	The head is superior to the pelvis.
anterior	toward the front	The eyes are anterior to the ears.
posterior	toward the back	The ears are posterior to the eyes.
ventral	toward the front	The stomach is ventral to the spine.
dorsal	toward the back	The spine is dorsal to the stomach.
medial	toward the midline of the body	The heart is medial to the arm.
lateral	further from the midline of the body	The arm is lateral to the chest.
proximal	closer to the trunk	The knee is proximal to the ankle.
distal	away from the trunk	The ankle is distal to the knee.

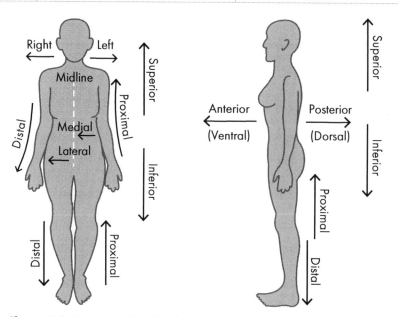

Figure 4.2. Anatomy Terminology

BODY CAVITIES

The internal structure of the human body is organized into compartments called **cavities**, which are separated by membranes. There are two main cavities in the human body: the dorsal cavity and the ventral cavity (both named for their relative positions).

The **dorsal cavity** is further divided into the **cranial cavity**, which holds the brain, and the **spinal cavity**, which surrounds the spine. The two sections of the dorsal cavity are continuous with each other. Both sections are lined by the **meninges**, a three-layered membrane that protects the brain and spinal cord.

The **ventral cavity** houses the majority of the body's organs. It also can be further divided into smaller cavities. The **thoracic cavity** holds the heart and lungs, the **abdominal cavity** holds the digestive organs and kidneys, and the **pelvic cavity** holds the bladder and reproductive organs. Both the abdominal and pelvic cavities are enclosed by a membrane called the **peritoneum**.

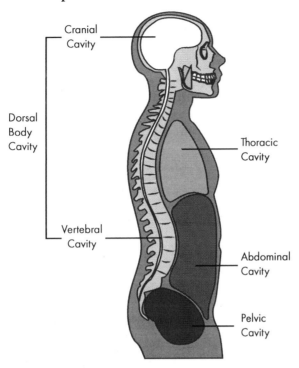

Figure 4.3. Body Cavities

PRACTICE QUESTIONS

1. Which term means *above* anatomically?
   A) anterior
   B) posterior
   C) superior
   D) medial

2. Where is the wrist located relative to the elbow?
   A) distal
   B) proximal
   C) anterior
   D) posterior

The Respiratory System
STRUCTURE AND FUNCTION OF THE RESPIRATORY SYSTEM

Mammalian cells require oxygen for glucose metabolism and release carbon dioxide as a byproduct. This process requires constant gas exchange between the human body and the environment to replenish the oxygen supply and remove carbon dioxide. This exchange is accomplished through the efforts of the **respiratory system**, in which powerful muscles force oxygen-rich air into the lungs and carbon dioxide-rich air out of the body.

Gas exchange takes place in the **lungs**. Humans have two lungs, a right and a left, with the right being slightly larger than the left due to the heart's placement in the left side of the chest cavity. The right lung has three **lobes**, and the left has two. The lungs are surrounded by a thick membrane called the **pleura**.

Air enters the body through the mouth or nasal cavity and passes through the **trachea** (sometimes called the windpipe) and into the two bronchi, each of which leads to one lung. Within the lung, the bronchi branch into smaller passageways called **bronchioles** and then terminate in sac-like structures called **alveoli**, which is where gas exchange between the air and the capillaries occurs. The large surface area of the alveoli allows for efficient exchange of gases through diffusion (movement of particles from areas of high to low concentration). Alveoli are covered in a layer of **surfactant**, which lubricates the sacs and prevents the lungs from collapsing.

HELPFUL HINT

In anatomy, the terms *right* and *left* are used with respect to the subject, not the observer.

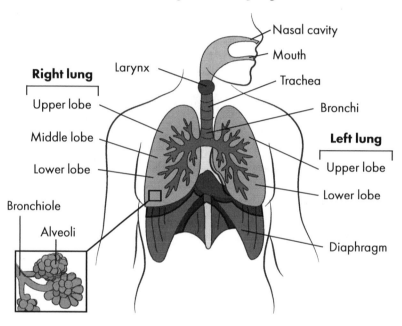

Figure 4.4. The Respiratory System

The heart pumps deoxygenated blood into the lungs via the **pulmonary artery**. This blood is oxygenated in the alveoli and then delivered back into the heart by the **pulmonary veins** for distribution to the body.

The **diaphragm** contributes to the activity of ventilation—the process of inhalation and exhalation. The contraction of the diaphragm creates a vacuum, forcing air into the lungs. Relaxation of the diaphragm compresses the lungs, forcing carbon dioxide-enriched gas out in exhalation. The amount of air breathed in and out is the **tidal volume**, and the **residual capacity** is the small volume of air left in the lungs after exhalation.

QUICK REVIEW

How might measuring tidal volume and residual capacity help evaluate respiratory health?

PATHOLOGIES OF THE RESPIRATORY SYSTEM

The body's critical and constant need for the exchange of carbon dioxide for oxygen makes the pulmonary system a locus of many serious diseases. Lung diseases that result in the continual restriction of airflow are known as **chronic obstructive pulmonary disease (COPD)**. These include **emphysema**, which is the destruction of lung tissues, and **asthma**, in which the airways are compromised due to a dysfunctional immune response. The main causes of COPD are smoking and air pollution, but genetic factors can also influence the severity of the disease.

The system is also prone to **respiratory tract infections**, with upper respiratory tract infections affecting air inputs in the nose and throat and lower respiratory tract infections affecting the lungs and their immediate pulmonary inputs. Viral infections of the respiratory system include influenza and the common cold; bacterial infections include tuberculosis and pertussis (whooping cough). **Pneumonia**, which affects alveoli, is a bacterial or viral infection that is often seen in people whose respiratory system has been weakened by other conditions.

PRACTICE QUESTIONS

3. Which of the following structures are small air sacs that function as the site of gas exchange in the lungs?

A) capillaries

B) bronchi

C) alveoli

D) cilia

4. Which of the following conditions is caused by an immune response?

A) COPD

B) influenza

C) asthma

D) emphysema

The Cardiovascular System

STRUCTURE OF BLOOD

The cardiovascular system circulates **blood**, which carries nutrients, waste products, hormones, and other important substances throughout the body. **Plasma** (also called blood plasma) is the liquid part of the blood. Elements suspended or dissolved in the plasma include gases, electrolytes, carbohydrates, fats, proteins, clotting factors, and waste products.

Red blood cells (RBCs) transport oxygen throughout the body. RBCs contain **hemoglobin**, a large molecule with iron atoms that bind to oxygen. **White blood cells (WBCs)** fight infection. **Platelets** (also called thrombocytes) gather at sites of damage in blood vessels as part of the blood-clotting process.

Blood groups (also called blood types) are determined by the presence of **antigens**, proteins that activate antibodies. Each blood group produces specific antibodies that

HELPFUL HINT

Thrombocytopenia is an abnormally low level of platelets.

attach to antigens on RBCs. The **ABO blood group** is defined by the presence or absence of A antigens and B antigens.

Table 4.2. The ABO Blood Groups

Blood Type	Antigens on RBC	Antibodies in Plasma
A	A antigens	anti-B antibodies
B	B antigens	anti-A antibodies
O	no antigens	anti-A and anti-B antibodies
AB	A and B antigens	no antibodies

HELPFUL HINT

Pregnant patients who are Rh-negative receive a shot that prevents their body from producing anti-Rh antibodies. This protects the fetus from hemolytic disease.

The Rh blood group is defined by the presence of **Rh factor**, an antigen also called the D antigen. The blood type **Rh-positive** has Rh factor antigens on RBCs; the blood type **Rh-negative** does not have Rh factor antigens on RBCs. In **hemolytic disease of the newborn**, anti-Rh antibodies in an Rh-negative mother attack the RBCs of her Rh-positive fetus.

THE COAGULATION PROCESS

Hemostasis is the process of stopping blood loss from a damaged blood vessel. Blood loss is stopped through **coagulation**, the process of turning liquid blood into a semisolid clot composed of platelets and red blood cells held together by the protein **fibrin**.

The process of coagulation is a complex cascade of reactions involving proteins called **clotting factors**.

HELPFUL HINT

Most clotting factors are designated by roman numerals. These numerals give the order in which factors were discovered, not the order in which they are activated.

- Platelet aggregation is initiated by the exposure to **von Willebrand factor (vW)** and **tissue factor (TF)**.

- During coagulation, the protein **fibrinogen** (factor I) is converted to fibrin by the enzyme **thrombin** (factor IIa).

- **Prothrombin** (factor II) is a precursor to thrombin.

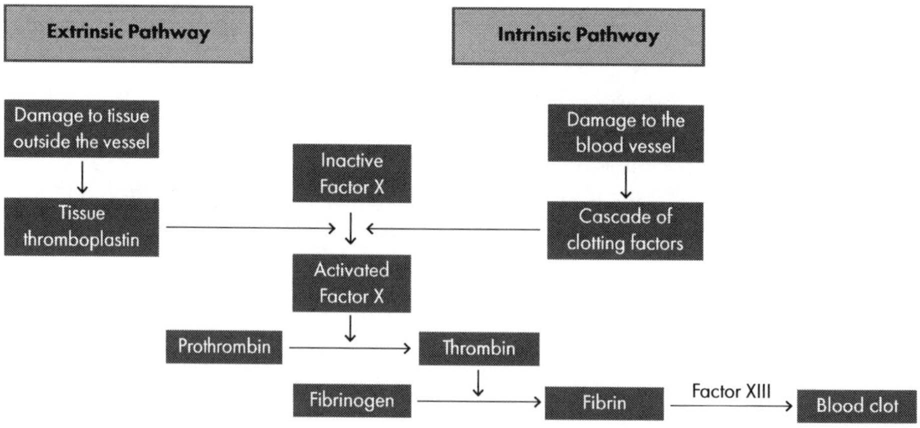

Figure 4.5. Clotting Cascade

5. What function do red blood cells perform in the human body?

    A) fight infection

    B) transport oxygen

    C) hydrate cells

    D) carry nutrients

6. Von Willebrand disease is caused by low levels or poor quality of von Willebrand factor. What signs and symptoms would a patient with von Willebrand disease likely have?

    A) nosebleeds

    B) rapid heartbeat

    C) trouble breathing

    D) headache

STRUCTURE AND FUNCTION OF THE CARDIOVASCULAR SYSTEM

Blood is circulated by a muscular organ called the **heart**. The circulatory system includes two closed loops. In the pulmonary loop, deoxygenated blood leaves the heart and travels to the lungs, where it loses carbon dioxide and becomes rich in oxygen. The oxygenated blood then returns to the heart, which pumps it through the systemic loop. The systemic loop delivers oxygen to the rest of the body and returns deoxygenated blood to

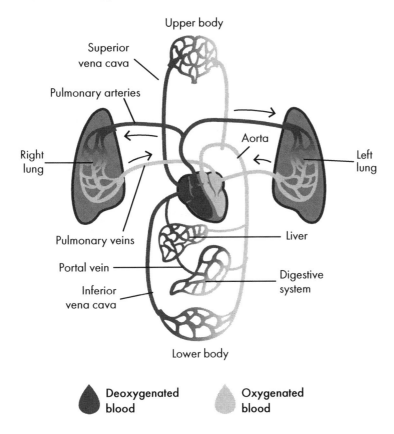

Figure 4.6. Circulatory System

the heart. The pumping action of the heart is regulated primarily by two neurological nodes, the **sinoatrial** and **atrioventricular nodes**, whose electrical activity sets the rhythm of the heart.

Deoxygenated blood from the body enters the heart via the **right atrium**. It then passes through the **tricuspid** valve into the **right ventricle** and is pumped out to the lungs. Oxygenated blood returns from the lungs into the **left atrium**. It then passes through the **mitral valve** into the **left ventricle** and is pumped out to the body through the **aorta**. The contraction of the heart during this process is called **systole**, and the relaxation of the heart is **diastole**.

Blood is carried through the body in a system of blood vessels. Oxygenated blood leaves the heart in large vessels called **arteries**, which branch into smaller and smaller vessels. The smallest vessels, **capillaries**, are where the exchange of molecules between blood and cells takes place. Deoxygenated blood returns to the heart in **veins**.

HELPFUL HINT

The pulmonary veins are the only veins in the human body that carry oxygenated blood.

Blood leaves the heart to travel to the body through the **aorta**; in the lower body, the aorta branches into the **iliac arteries**. Deoxygenated blood returns to the heart from the body via the **superior vena cava** (upper body) and **inferior vena cava** (lower body). Blood then leaves the heart again to travel to the lungs through the **pulmonary arteries**, and returns from the lungs via the **pulmonary veins**.

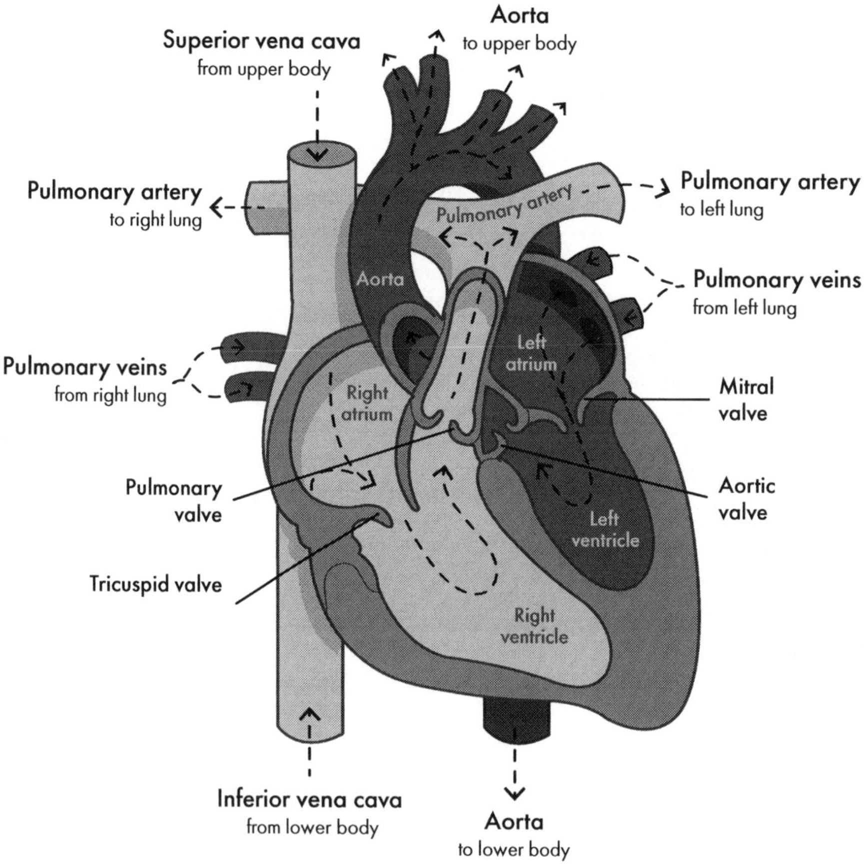

Figure 4.7. The Heart

THE LYMPHATIC SYSTEM

The **lymphatic system** is an open circulatory system that functions alongside the cardiovascular system. It facilitates the movement of substances between cells and the blood by removing interstitial fluid (the fluid between cells). It also plays an important role in the immune system by circulating white blood cells. The system is composed of **lymphatic vessels** that carry **lymph**, a clear fluid containing lymphocytes and waste products. Lymph passes through **lymph nodes**, which are collections of tissue rich in white blood cells that filter out harmful substances such as pathogens and cell waste. The lymph is then returned to the circulatory system through the veins near the heart.

PATHOLOGIES OF THE CARDIOVASCULAR SYSTEM

The cardiovascular system is subject to a number of pathologies. In a **heart attack**, blood flow to part of the heart is stopped, causing damage to the heart muscle. An irregular heartbeat, called an **arrhythmia**, is caused by disruptions with the electrical signals in the heart. Many arrhythmias can be treated—with a pacemaker, for example—or do not cause any symptoms.

Problems with blood vessels include **atherosclerosis**, in which white blood cells and plaque build up in arteries, and **hypertension**, or high blood pressure. In a stroke, blood flow is blocked in the brain, resulting in damage to brain cells.

PRACTICE QUESTIONS

7. The mitral valve transports blood between which of the following two regions of the heart?

   A) aorta and left atrium

   B) aorta and right atrium

   C) right atrium and right ventricle

   D) left atrium and left ventricle

8. Which of the following supplies blood to the lower body?

   A) superior vena cava

   B) inferior vena cava

   C) iliac artery

   D) aortic arch

9. Which of the following electrically signals the heart to pump?

   A) sinoatrial node

   B) aorta

   C) mitral valve

   D) left ventricle

The Nervous System

The nervous system is made up of two distinct parts: the central nervous system (brain and spinal cord) and the peripheral nervous system. However, the fundamental physiological principles underlying both systems are similar. In both systems, **neurons** communicate electrically and chemically with one another along pathways. These pathways allow the nervous system as a whole to conduct its incredibly broad array of functions, from motor control and sensory perception to complex thinking and emotions.

NERVE CELLS

Neurons, a.k.a. nerve cells, have several key anatomical features that contribute to their specialized functions. These cells typically contain an **axon**, a long projection from the cell that sends information over a distance. These cells also have **dendrites**, which are long, branching extensions of the cell that receive information from neighboring cells. The number of dendrites and the extent of their branching varies widely, distinguishing the various types of these cells.

Neurons and nerve cells do not touch; instead, communication occurs across a specialized gap called a **synapse**. The chemicals that facilitate communication across synapses are known as **neurotransmitters**, and include serotonin and dopamine. Communication occurs when electrical signals cause the **axon terminal** to release neurotransmitters.

Nerve cells are accompanied by glia, or supporting cells, that surround the cell and provide support, protection, and nutrients. In the peripheral nervous system, the primary glial cell is a **Schwann cell**. Schwann cells secrete a fatty substance called **myelin** that wraps around the neuron and allows much faster transmission of the electrical signal the neuron is sending. Gaps in the myelin sheath are called nodes of Ranvier.

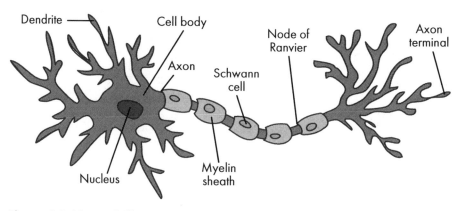

Figure 4.8. Nerve Cell

THE CENTRAL NERVOUS SYSTEM

The central nervous system, which includes the brain and spinal cord, is responsible for arguably the body's most complex and abstract functions, including cognition, emotion, and behavioral regulation. The brain is divided into six general regions:

- **cerebrum**: the largest part of the brain; responsible for voluntary movement, language, learning, and memory
- **diencephalon**: includes the thalamus, hypothalamus, and pineal body; relays sensory information and controls some automatic functions of the peripheral nervous system

- **mesencephalon** (midbrain): processes hearing and visual information; maintains sleep/wake cycles and temperature
- **pons**: controls many involuntary processes, including respiration, bladder control, and sleep; also responsible for facial movements and eye movement
- **cerebellum**: responsible for motor control and motor learning
- **medulla oblongata**: controls involuntary processes of the cardiac and respiratory systems; responsible for reflexes such as sneezing and vomiting

The cerebrum and cerebellum are further broken down into **lobes** that each carry out a broad common function. For example, in the cerebrum, the processing of visual information occurs in the **occipital lobe,** and the **temporal lobe** is involved in language comprehension and emotional associations.

In addition to its organization by lobes and structures, regions of the brain are also designated by myelination status: **white matter** regions are myelinated and **gray matter** regions are unmyelinated. Brain structures in the cerebral cortex (the outermost brain layer) form a convoluted pattern of **gyri** (ridges) and **sulci** (valleys) that maximize the ratio of surface area to volume.

HELPFUL HINT

Alzheimer's disease, which causes dementia, is the result of damaged neurons in the cerebral cortex, the area of the brain responsible for higher order functions like information processing and language.

THE PERIPHERAL NERVOUS SYSTEM

The peripheral nervous system, which includes all the nerve cells outside the brain and spinal cord, has one main function and that is to communicate between the CNS and the rest of the body.

The peripheral nervous system is further divided into two systems. The **automatic nervous system** (ANS) is the part of the peripheral nervous system that controls involuntary bodily functions such as digestion, respiration, and heart rate. The autonomic nervous system is further broken down into the sympathetic nervous system and parasympathetic nervous system.

The **sympathetic nervous system** is responsible for the body's reaction to stress and induces a "fight or flight" response to stimuli. For instance, if an individual is frightened, the sympathetic nervous system increases the person's heart rate and blood pressure to prepare that person to either fight or flee.

In contrast, the **parasympathetic nervous system** is stimulated by the body's need for rest or recovery. The parasympathetic nervous system responds by decreasing heart rate, blood pressure, and muscular activation when a person is getting ready for activities such as sleeping or digesting food. For example, the body activates the parasympathetic nervous system after a person eats a large meal, which is why that individual may then feel sluggish.

The second part of the peripheral nervous system, called the **somatic nervous system**, controls sensory information and motor control. Generally, nerve cells can be divided into two types. **Afferent** (sensory) cells relay messages to the central nervous system, and **efferent** (motor) cells carry messages to the muscles. In the motor nervous system, signals from the brain travel down the spinal cord before exiting and communicating with motor nerve cells, which synapse on muscle fibers at **neuromuscular junctions**. Because individuals can control the movement of skeletal muscle, this part of the nervous system is considered voluntary.

HELPFUL HINT

The "fight or flight" reaction includes accelerated breathing and heart rate, dilation of blood vessels in muscles, release of energy molecules for use by muscles, relaxation of the bladder, and slowing or stopping movement in the upper digestive tract.

Some **reflexes**, or automatic response to stimuli, are able to occur rapidly by bypassing the brain altogether. In a **reflex arc**, a signal is sent from the peripheral nervous system to the spinal cord, which then sends a signal directly to a motor cells, causing movement.

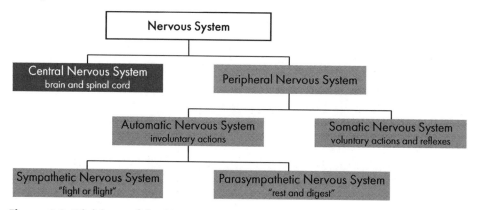

Figure 4.9. Divisions of the Nervous System

PATHOLOGIES OF THE NERVOUS SYSTEM

The nervous system can be affected by a number of degenerative diseases that result from the gradual breakdown of nervous tissue. These include:

- **Parkinson's disease**: caused by cell death in the basal ganglia; characterized by gradual loss of motor function

- **multiple sclerosis (MS)**: caused by damage to the myelin sheath; characterized by muscle spasms and weakness, numbness, loss of coordination, and blindness

- **amyotrophic lateral sclerosis (ALS)**: caused by the death of neurons that control voluntary muscle movement; characterized by muscle stiffness, twitches, and weakness

- **Alzheimer's disease**: caused by damaged neurons in the cerebral cortex; characterized by memory loss, confusion, mood swings, and problems with language

The nervous system is also susceptible to infections, some of which can be life threatening. **Meningitis** is inflammation of the meninges, the protective membrane that surrounds the brain and spinal cord, and **encephalitis** is inflammation of the brain. Both conditions can be caused by viral or bacterial pathogens.

Epileptic seizures are brief episodes caused by disturbed or overactive nerve cell activity in the brain. Seizures range widely in severity and may include confusion, convulsions, and loss of consciousness. They have many causes, including tumors, infections, head injuries, and medications.

PRACTICE QUESTIONS

10. Which part of the nervous system controls only voluntary action?

    A) the peripheral nervous system

    B) the somatic nervous system

    C) the sympathetic nervous system

    D) the parasympathetic nervous system

The Gastrointestinal System

STRUCTURE AND FUNCTION OF THE GASTROINTESTINAL SYSTEM

Fueling the biological systems mentioned previously is the digestive system. The digestive system is essentially a continuous tube in which food is processed. During digestion, the body extracts necessary nutrients and biological fuels and isolates waste to be discarded.

The breakdown of food into its constituent parts begins as soon as it is put into the mouth. Enzymes in **saliva** such as salivary amylase begin breaking down food, particularly starch, as mastication helps prepare food for swallowing and subsequent digestion. Food from this point is formed into a **bolus** that travels down the esophagus, aided by a process called **peristalsis**, rhythmic contractions that move the partially digested food towards the stomach. Upon reaching the **stomach**, food encounters a powerful acid (composed mainly of hydrochloric acid), which aids the breakdown of food into its absorbable components.

The human body derives fuel primarily from three sources: proteins, sugars, and fats (lipids). Enzymes break proteins down into their constituent amino acids to produce new proteins for the body. Carbohydrates are broken down enzymatically if necessary and used for metabolism. Fats are broken down into constituent fatty acids and glycerol for a number of uses, including dense nutritional energy storage. Digestion of fat requires **bile** acids produced by the **liver**; bile is stored in the **gall bladder**.

The stomach produces a semifluid mass of partially digested food called **chyme** that passes into the **small intestine**, where nutrients are absorbed into the bloodstream. This absorption occurs through millions of finger-like projections known as **villi** that increase the surface area available for the absorption of nutrients.

HELPFUL HINT

The burning sensation called heartburn occurs when gastric acid from the stomach travels up the esophagus, often as a result of relaxation of the lower esophageal sphincter. This acid can damage the lining of the esophagus.

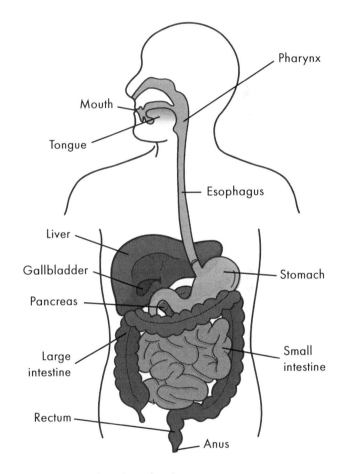

Figure 4.10. The Digestive System

The small intestine itself has three major segments. Proximal to the stomach is the **duodenum**, which combines digestive substances from the liver and pancreas; next is the **jejunum**, the primary site of nutrient absorption; finally, the **ileum** absorbs remaining nutrients and moves the remaining matter into the large intestine. The **large intestine** (also called the colon) absorbs water from the waste, which then passes into the **rectum** and out of the body through the **anus**.

PATHOLOGIES OF THE GASTROINTESTINAL SYSTEM

The digestive system is prone to several illnesses of varying severity. Commonly, gastro-intestinal distress is caused by an acute infection (bacterial or viral) affecting the lining of the digestive system. A resulting immune response triggers the body, as an adaptive measure, to void the contents of the digestive system in order to purge the infection. Chronic gastrointestinal disorders include **irritable bowel syndrome** (the causes of which are largely unknown) and **Crohn's disease**, an inflammatory bowel disorder with an immune-related etiology.

PRACTICE QUESTIONS

12. Where in the digestive tract are most of the nutrients absorbed?
   A) the small intestine
   B) the rectum
   C) the stomach
   D) the large intestine

13. Which of the following initiates the breakdown of carbohydrates?
   A) salivary amylase
   B) stomach acid
   C) bile salts
   D) peristalsis

The Skeletal System
STRUCTURE AND FUNCTION OF THE SKELETAL SYSTEM

The skeletal system is composed of tissue called **bone** that helps with movement, provides support for organs, and synthesizes blood cells. The outer layer of bone is composed of a matrix made of collagen and minerals that gives bones their strength and rigidity. The matrix is formed from functional units called **osteons** that include layers of compact bone called **lamellae**. The lamellae surround a cavity called the **Haversian canal**, which houses the bone's blood supply. These canals are in turn connected to the **periosteum**, the bone's outermost membrane, by another series of channels called **Volkmann's canals**.

Within osteons are blood cells called **osteoblasts**, mononucleate cells that produce bone tissue. When the bone tissue hardens around these cells, the cells are known as **osteocytes**, and the space they occupy within the bone tissue is known as **lacunae**. The lacunae are connected by a series of channels called **canaliculi**. **Osteoclasts**, a third type of bone cell, are responsible for breaking down bone tissue. They are located on the surface of bones and help balance the body's calcium levels by degrading bone to release stored calcium. The fourth type of bone cell, **lining cells** are flatted osteoblasts that protect the bone and also help balance calcium levels.

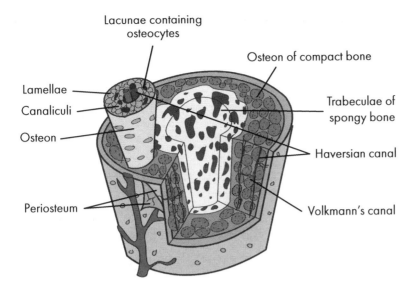

Figure 4.11. Bone Structure

Within the hard outer layer of bone is the spongy layer called **cancellous bone**, which is made up of support structures called **trabeculae**. Within this layer is the bone marrow, which houses cells that produce red blood cells in a process called **hematopoiesis**. Bone marrow also produces many of the lymphocytes that play an important role in the immune system.

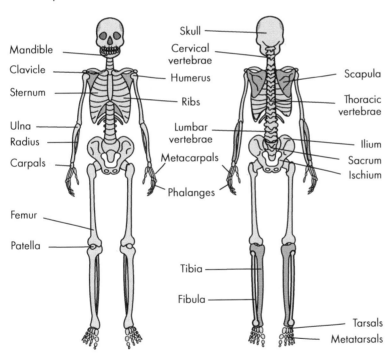

Figure 4.12. The Skeletal System

Bones are divided into four main categories. **Long bones**, such as the femur and humerus, are longer than they are wide. **Short bones**, in contrast, are wider than they are long. These include the clavicle and carpals. **Flat bones** are wide and flat, and usually provide protection. Examples of flat bones include the bones of the skull, pelvis, and rib cage. **Irregular bones**, as the name suggests, have an irregular shape that doesn't fit into the other categories. These bones include the vertebrae and bones of the jaw.

Bones are held together (articulated) at **joints** by connective tissue called **ligaments**. Joints can be classified based on the tissue that connects the bone. **Fibrous joints** are connected by dense, collagen-rich fibers, while **cartilaginous joints** are joined by special tissue called **hyaline cartilage**. Cartilage is more flexible than bone but denser than muscles. In addition to joining together bone, it also helps hold open passageways and provides support in structures like the nose and ears. The third type of joint, **synovial joints**, are joined by synovial fluid, which lubricates the joint and allows for movement. Bones are also joined to muscles by connective tissue called **tendons**.

Table 4.3. Types of Synovial Joints

Name	Movement	Found In
Hinge joint	movement through one plane of motion as flexion/extension	elbows, knees, fingers
Ball-and-socket joint	range of motion through multiple planes and rotation about an axis	hips, shoulders
Saddle joint	movement through multiple planes, but cannot rotate about an axis	thumbs
Gliding joint	sliding movement in the plane of the bones' surfaces	vertebrae, small bones in the wrists and ankles
Condyloid joint	movement through two planes as flexion/extension and abduction/adduction, but cannot rotate about an axis	wrists
Pivot joint	only movement is rotation about an axis	elbows, neck

PATHOLOGIES OF THE SKELETAL SYSTEM

Important pathologies of the skeletal system include **osteoporosis**, which occurs when minerals are leached from the bone, making bones more likely to break. Broken bones can also be caused by **brittle bone disease**, which results from a genetic defect that affects collagen production. Joint pain can be caused by **osteoarthritis**, which is the breakdown of cartilage in joints, and **rheumatoid arthritis**, which is an autoimmune disease that affects synovial membranes.

PRACTICE QUESTIONS

14. Which type of cell is responsible for the degradation of bone tissue?
    A) osteoclasts
    B) osteoblasts
    C) osteocytes
    D) lining cells

15. Which joint allows for the most freedom of movement?

A) fibrous joints

B) hinge joints

C) saddle joints

D) ball-and-socket joints

The Muscular System

TYPES OF MUSCLE

The muscular system is composed of **muscles** that move the body, support bodily functions, and circulate blood. The human body contains three types of muscles. **Skeletal muscles** are voluntarily controlled and attach to the skeleton to allow movement in the body. **Smooth muscles** are involuntary, meaning they cannot be consciously controlled. Smooth muscles are found in many organs and structures, including the esophagus, stomach, intestines, blood vessels, bladder, and bronchi. Finally, **cardiac muscles**, found only in the heart, are the involuntary muscles that contract the heart in order to pump blood through the body.

HELPFUL HINT

Some skeletal muscles, such as the diaphragm and those that control blinking, can be voluntarily controlled but usually operate involuntarily.

MUSCLE CELL STRUCTURE

The main structural unit of a muscle is the **sarcomere**. Sarcomeres are composed of a series of **muscle fibers**, which are elongated individual cells that stretch from one end of the muscle to the other. Within each fiber are hundreds of **myofibrils**, long strands within the cells that contain alternating layers of thin filaments made of the protein **actin** and thick filaments made of the protein **myosin**. Each of these proteins plays a role in muscle contraction and relaxation.

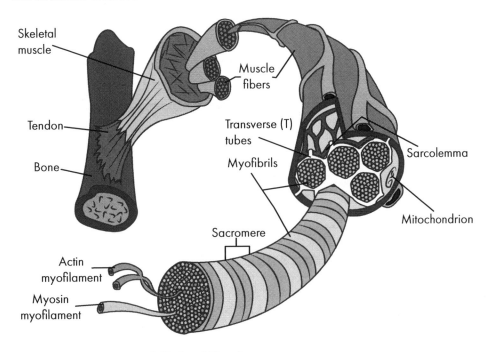

Figure 4.13. Structure of Skeletal Muscle

Muscle contraction is explained by the **sliding filament theory**. When the sarcomere is at rest, the thin filaments containing actin are found at both ends of the muscle, while the thick filaments containing myosin are found at the center. Myosin filaments contain "heads," which can attach and detach from actin filaments. The myosin attaches to actin and pulls the thin filaments to the center of the sarcomere, forcing the thin filaments to slide inward and causing the entire sarcomere to shorten, or contract, creating movement. The sarcomere can be broken down into zones that contain certain filaments.

- The **Z-line** separates the sarcomeres: a single sarcomere is the distance between two Z-lines.

- The **A-band** is the area of the sarcomere in which thick myosin filaments are found and does not shorten during muscular contraction.

- The **I-band** is the area in the sarcomere between the thick myosin filaments in which only thin actin filament is found.

- The **H-zone** is found between the actin filaments and contains only thick myosin filament.

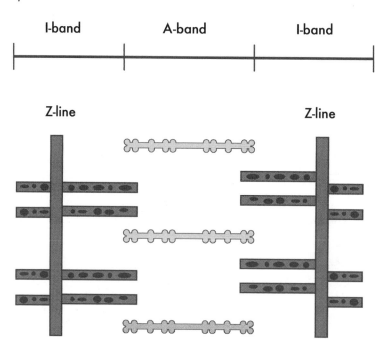

Figure 4.14. Sliding Filament Theory

PATHOLOGIES OF THE MUSCULAR SYSTEM

Injuries to muscle can impede movement and cause pain. When muscle fibers are over-stretched, the resulting **muscle strain** can cause pain, stiffness, and bruising. Muscle fibers can also be weakened by diseases, as with **muscular dystrophy** (MD). MD is a genetically inherited condition that results in progressive muscle wasting, which limits movement and can cause respiratory and cardiovascular difficulties.

HELPFUL HINT

Overstretching a ligament is called a *sprain*.

16. Which type of muscle is responsible for voluntary movement in the body?

    A) cardiac

    B) visceral

    C) smooth

    D) skeletal

17. Which of the following causes a muscle strain?

    A) a lack of available energy

    B) the inability of muscle fibers to contract

    C) detachment of the ligament from the bone

    D) overstretching of muscle fibers

The Immune System

The human immune system protects the body against bacteria and viruses that cause disease. The system is composed of two parts. The **innate** system includes nonspecific defenses that work against a wide range of infectious agents. This system includes both physical barriers that keep out foreign particles and organisms along with specific cells that attack invaders that move past barriers. The second part of the immune system is the **adaptive** immune system, which "learns" to respond only to specific invaders.

Table 4.4. Lines of Defense in the Immune System

1. External barriers	skin, enzymes, mucus, earwax, native bacteria
2. The innate response	inflammation, neutrophils (a white blood cell), antimicrobial peptides, natural killer lymphocytes, interferon
3. The adaptive response	helper T cells, cytotoxic T cells, B cells, memory B cells

THE INNATE IMMUNE SYSTEM

The first line of defense in the immune system are barriers to entry. The most prominent is the **skin**, which leaves few openings for an infection-causing agent to enter. Bodily orifices exhibit other methods for preventing infection. The mouth is saturated with native bacteria that dominate the resources in the microenvironment, making it inhospitable to invading bacteria. In addition, enzymes in the mouth create a hostile environment for foreign organisms. The urethra flushes away potentially invasive microorganisms mechanically through the outflow of urine, while the vagina maintains a consistently low pH, deterring potential infections. The eyes and nose constantly produce and flush away tears and **mucus**, which trap pathogens before they can replicate and infect. Similarly, **earwax** serves as an additional barrier to entry.

Pathogens do occasionally breach these barriers and arrive within the body, where they attempt to replicate and cause an infection. When this occurs, the body mounts a number of nonspecific responses. The body's initial response is **inflammation**: infected cells release signaling molecules indicating that an infection has occurred, which causes increased blood flow to the area. This increase in blood flow includes the increased

HELPFUL HINT

Phagocytosis occurs when a cell completely surrounds a particle to form an enclosed vesicle. The particle can then be broken down either for nutrients or to neutralize a threat. Cells in the immune system that use phagocytosis are called macrophages.

presence of **white blood cells**, also called **leukocytes**. The most common type of leukocyte found at sites of inflammation are **neutrophils**, which engulf and destroy invaders.

Other innate responses include **antimicrobial peptides**, which destroy bacteria by interfering with the functions of their membranes or DNA, and **natural killer lymphocytes**, which respond to virus-infected cells. Because they can recognize damaged cells with the presence of antibodies, they are important in early defense against bacterial infection. In addition, infected cells may release **interferon**, which causes nearby cells to increase their defenses.

Table 4.5. Types of White Blood Cells

Type of Cell	Name of Cell	Role	Innate or Adaptive	Prevalence
Granulocytes	Neutrophil	First responders that quickly migrate to the site of infections to destroy bacterial invaders	Innate	Very common
	Eosinophil	Attack multicellular parasites	Innate	Rare
	Basophil	Large cell responsible for inflammatory reactions, including allergies	Innate	Very rare
Lymphocyte	B cells	Respond to antigens by releasing antibodies	Adaptive	Common
	T cells	Respond to antigens by destroying invaders and infected cells	Adaptive	
	Natural killer cells	Destroy virus-infected cells and tumor cells	Innate and adaptive	
Monocyte	Macrophage	Engulf and destroy microbes, foreign substances, and cancer cells	Innate and adaptive	Rare

THE ADAPTIVE IMMUNE SYSTEM

The adaptive immune system is able to recognize molecules called **antigens** on the surface of pathogens to which the system has previously been exposed. Antigens are displayed on the surface of cells by the **major histocompatibility complex** (MHC), which can display either "self" proteins from their own cells or proteins from pathogens. In an **antigen-presenting cell**, the MHC on the cell's surface displays a particular antigen, which is recognized by **helper T cells**. These cells produce a signal (cytokines) that activates **cytotoxic T cells**, which then destroy any cell that displays the antigen.

The presence of antigens also activates **B cells**, which rapidly multiply to create **plasma cells**, which in turn release **antibodies**. Antibodies will bind only to specific antigens, and in turn result in the destruction of the infected cell. Some interfere directly with the function of the cell, while others draw the attention of macrophages. **Memory**

HELPFUL HINT

Memory B cells are the underlying mechanisms behind vaccines, which introduce a harmless version of a pathogen into the body to active the body's adaptive immune response.

B cells are created during infection. These cells "remember" the antigen that their parent cells responded to, allowing them to respond more quickly if the infection appears again.

Together, T and B cells are known as **lymphocytes**. T cells are produced in the thymus, while B cells mature in bone marrow. These cells circulate through the lymphatic system.

PATHOLOGIES OF THE IMMUNE SYSTEM

The immune system itself can be pathological. The immune system of individuals with an **autoimmune disease** will attack healthy tissues, as is the case in lupus, psoriasis, and multiple sclerosis. The immune system may also overreact to harmless particles, a condition known as an **allergy**. Some infections will attack the immune system itself. **Human immunodeficiency virus (HIV)** attacks helper T cells, eventually causing **acquired immunodeficiency syndrome (AIDS)**, which allows opportunistic infections to overrun the body.

PRACTICE QUESTIONS

18. Which of the following is NOT part of the innate immune system?

A) interferon

B) neutrophils

C) antibodies

D) natural killer lymphocytes

19. Which of the following is NOT considered a nonspecific defense of the innate immune system?

A) the skin

B) inflammation

C) antimicrobial peptides

D) antibody production

The Endocrine System
STRUCTURE AND FUNCTION OF THE ENDOCRINE SYSTEM

The endocrine system is composed of a network of organs called **glands** that produce signaling chemicals called **hormones**. These hormones are released by glands into the bloodstream and then travel to the other tissues and organs whose functions they regulate. When they reach their target, hormones bond to a specific receptor on cell membranes, which affects the machinery of the cell. Hormones play an important role in regulating almost all bodily functions, including digestion, respiration, sleep, stress, growth, development, reproduction, and immune response.

Much of the action of the endocrine system runs through the **hypothalamus**, which is highly integrated into the nervous system. The hypothalamus receives signals from the brain and in turn will release hormones that regulate both other endocrine organs and important metabolic processes. Other endocrine glands include the pineal, pituitary, thyroid, parathyroid, thymus, and adrenal glands.

Organs from other systems, including the reproductive and digestive systems, can also secrete hormones, and thus are considered part of the endocrine system. The reproductive organs in both males (testes) and females (ovaries and placenta) release important hormones, as do the pancreas, liver, and stomach.

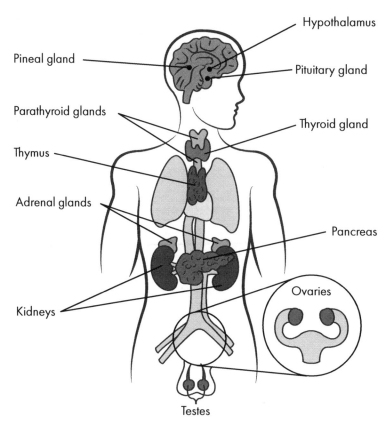

Figure 4.15. The Endocrine System

Table 4.6. Endocrine Glands		
Gland	**Regulates**	**Hormones Produced**
Pineal gland	circadian rhythms (the sleep/wake cycle)	melatonin
Pituitary gland	growth, blood pressure, reabsorption of water by the kidneys, temperature, pain relief, and some reproductive functions related to pregnancy and childbirth	human growth hormone (HGH), thyroid-stimulating hormone (TSH), prolactin (PRL), luteinizing hormone (LH), follicle-stimulating hormone (FSH), oxytocin, antidiuretic hormone (ADH)
Hypothalamus	pituitary function and metabolic processes including body temperature, hunger, thirst, and circadian rhythms	thyrotropin-releasing hormone (TRH), dopamine, growth-hormone-releasing hormone (GHRH), gonadotropin-releasing hormone (GnRH), oxytocin, vasopressin

Gland	Regulates	Hormones Produced
Thyroid gland	energy use and protein synthesis	thyroxine (T4), triiodothyronine (T3), calcitonin
Parathyroid	calcium and phosphate levels	parathyroid hormone (PTH)
Adrenal glands	"fight or flight" response, regulation of salt and blood volume	epinephrine, norepinephrine, cortisol, androgens
Pancreas	blood sugar levels and metabolism	insulin, glucagon, somatostatin
Testes	maturation of sex organs, secondary sex characteristics	androgens (e.g., testosterone)
Ovaries	maturation of sex organs, secondary sex characteristics, pregnancy, childbirth, and lactation	progesterone, estrogens
Placenta	gestation and childbirth	progesterone, estrogens, human chorionic gonadotropin, human placental lactogen

PATHOLOGIES OF THE ENDOCRINE SYSTEM

Disruption of hormone production in specific endocrine glands can lead to disease. An inability to produce insulin results in uncontrolled blood glucose levels, a condition called **diabetes**. Over- or underactive glands can lead to conditions like **hypothyroidism**, which is characterized by slow metabolism, and hyperparathyroidism, which can lead to osteoporosis. Tumors on endocrine glands can also damage the functioning of a wide variety of bodily systems.

PRACTICE QUESTIONS

20. Which gland in the endocrine system is responsible for regulating blood glucose levels?

A) adrenal

B) testes

C) pineal

D) pancreas

21. Damage to the parathyroid would most likely affect which of the following?

A) stress levels

B) bone density

C) secondary sex characteristics

D) circadian rhythms

The Genitourinary System

The **urinary system** excretes water and waste from the body and is crucial for maintaining the body's electrolyte balance (the balance of water and salt in the blood). Because many organs function as part of both the reproductive and urinary systems, the two are sometimes referred to collectively as the **genitourinary system.**

HELPFUL HINT

A normal human kidney contains around one million nephrons.

The main organs of the urinary system are the **kidneys,** which filter waste from the blood; maintain the electrolyte balance in the blood; and regulate blood volume, pressure, and pH. The kidneys also function as an endocrine organ and release several important hormones. These include **renin,** which regulates blood pressure, and **calcitriol,** the active form of vitamin D. The kidney is divided into two regions: the **renal cortex,** which is the outermost layer, and the **renal medulla,** which is the inner layer.

The functional unit of the kidney is the **nephron,** which is a series of looping tubes that filter electrolytes, metabolic waste, and other water-soluble waste molecules from the blood. These wastes include **urea,** which is a nitrogenous byproduct of protein catabolism, and **uric acid,** a byproduct of nucleic acid metabolism. Together, these waste products are excreted from the body in **urine.**

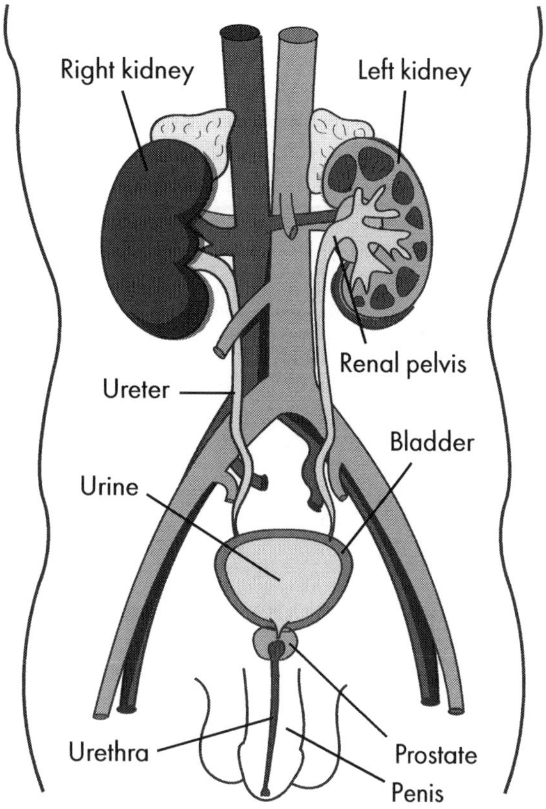

Figure 4.16. Male Genitourinary System

Filtration begins in a network of capillaries called a **glomerulus** which is located in the renal cortex of each kidney. This waste is then funneled into **collecting ducts** in the renal medulla. From the collecting ducts, urine passes through the **renal pelvis** and then through two long tubes called **ureters.**

The two ureters drain into the urinary bladder, which holds up to 1000 milliliters of liquid. The bladder exit is controlled by two sphincters, both of which must open for urine to pass. The internal sphincter is made of smooth involuntary muscle, while the external sphincter can be voluntarily controlled. In males, the external sphincter also closes to prevent movement of seminal fluid into the bladder during sexual activity. (A sphincter is a circular muscle that controls movement of substances through passageways. Sphincters are found throughout the human body, including the bladder, esophagus, and capillaries.)

Urine exits the bladder through the **urethra.** In males, the urethra goes through the penis and also carries semen. In females, the much-shorter urethra ends just above the vaginal opening.

PRACTICE QUESTIONS

22. Which of the following is the outermost layer of the kidney?

A) renal cortex

B) renal medulla

C) renal pelvis

D) nephron

23. Which of the following organs holds urine before it passes into the urethra?

A) prostate

B) kidney

C) ureter

D) urinary bladder

1. **C) is correct.** Superior means that something is above a reference point.

2. **A) is correct.** The wrist is distal, or further from the trunk, than the elbow.

3. **C) is correct.** The alveoli are sacs found at the terminal end of each bronchiole in the lungs and are the site of gas exchange with the blood.

4. **C) is correct.** Asthma is a negative reaction of the body to otherwise harmless particles.

5. **B) is correct.** Red blood cells (RBCs) carry oxygen throughout the body so it can be absorbed into cells and used for cellular respiration. Oxygen is carried on hemoglobin, an iron-containing protein found in RBCs.

6. **A) is correct.** People with von Willebrand disease will bleed easily and for longer periods of time. Symptoms range from easy bruising and nosebleeds to life-threatening hemorrhages following trauma or surgery.

7. **D) is correct.** These two structures form a junction at the mitral valve.

8. **C) is correct.** The iliac artery receives blood from the aorta to supply blood to the lower body.

9. **A) is correct.** The sinoatrial and atrioventricular nodes electrically stimulate the heart to pump.

10. **B) is correct.** The somatic nervous system controls voluntary actions.

11. **B) is correct.** Dendrites receive information in nerve cells.

12. **A) is correct.** Most nutrients are absorbed by the small intestine.

13. **A) is correct.** Salivary amylase in the mouth begins the breakdown of carbohydrates.

14. **A) is correct.** Osteoclasts break down and absorb bone tissue.

15. **D) is correct.** Ball-and-socket joints allow for the most freedom of movement.

16. **D) is correct.** Skeletal muscles are attached to the skeletal system and are controlled voluntarily.

17. **D) is correct.** A muscle strain is caused by the overstretching of muscle fibers, resulting in tearing of the muscle.

18. **C) is correct.** Antibodies are part of the body's adaptive immune system and only respond to specific pathogens.

19. **D) is correct.** Antibodies are produced by B-cells as part of an adaptive immune response.

20. **D) is correct.** The pancreas releases insulin and glucagon, which regulate glucose levels in the blood.

21. **B) is correct.** The parathyroid controls calcium and phosphate levels, which are maintained by producing and reabsorbing bone tissue.

22. **A) is correct.** The outermost layer of the kidney is the renal cortex.

23. **D) is correct.** The urinary bladder holds urine before it passes to the urethra to be excreted.

FIVE: PRACTICE TEST

Reading

Directions: Read the passage, and then answer the questions that follow.

The following passage refers to questions 1–6.

The endocrine system is made up of glands—such as the parathyroid, thyroid, pituitary, and adrenals—that produce hormones. Men and women have different reproductive glands: men have testes and women have ovaries. The pituitary gland serves as the "master gland" of the endocrine system.

The endocrine system's function is to produce and distribute hormones. Endocrine glands release hormones into the bloodstream, where they are carried to other tissues or organs. When the hormones reach other tissues, they catalyze certain chemical reactions, stimulating various processes or activities. For instance, hormones are responsible for important bodily processes such as puberty and menstruation. Hormones are also released in humans in moments of fear or anxiety and can trigger the fight-or-flight response. The endocrine system is the primary source of a wide range of physiological activities and is sometimes referred to as the "hardworking chemical control center" of the human body.

1. What is the author's primary purpose in writing this essay?

   A) to warn people about the dangers of hormonal imbalance

   B) to persuade people to take care of their endocrine glands

   C) to advise people about different hormones and what they do

   D) to inform people about the endocrine system's parts and functions

2. Which of the following statements can be considered a statement of FACT according to the content offered in the paragraphs above?

   A) The endocrine system is the most important system in the human body.

   B) The endocrine system is the only "chemical control center in the body."

   C) The endocrine system only has one organ: the pancreas.

   D) The endocrine system stimulates reactions in the body by releasing hormones.

3. What is the best summary of the passage?

A) The endocrine system controls hormones that stimulate processes in the body.

B) Endocrine glands differ in men and women.

C) The pituitary gland is the "master gland" of the endocrine system.

D) Hormones are responsible for puberty and menstruation.

4. According to the passage, what is true about hormones?

A) They are only secreted by the pancreas.

B) They can help trigger fight-or-flight responses.

C) They almost always cause negative reactions.

D) Their sole purpose is to stimulate reproductive activities.

5. According to the passage, what serves as the major organ associated with the endocrine system?

A) the pituitary gland

B) the testicles

C) the ovaries

D) the spinal cord

6. What is the meaning of the word *stimulating* in the second paragraph?

A) to make something happen

B) to reproduce something

C) to create fear or anxiety

D) to destroy or diminish a tissue

The following passage refers to questions 7–12.

Every medical professional should understand the root causes and potential effects of hypoglycemia because it can actually be a matter of life or death for a patient with diabetes. Hypoglycemia—which literally means low (*hypo*) blood sugar (*glycemia*)—is one of the most common medical emergencies for patients who have diabetes. Hypoglycemia can occur when a patient either takes too much insulin or has not consumed enough sugar. At other times, hypoglycemia stems from overexertion. A person can even become hypoglycemic if they vomit an important meal, depriving the body of the sugar and nutrients it needs to stay balanced.

Any medical professional interacting with diabetic patients should know the telltale signs of hypoglycemia. When a diabetic patient's blood sugar plummets, their mental state becomes altered. This can lead to unconsciousness or, in more severe cases, a diabetic coma and/or brain damage. If you notice the rapid onset of nervousness or anxiety, shakiness, and/or profuse sweating in someone with diabetes, you will likely need to help administer glucose to them as soon as possible (as long as they are conscious enough to swallow). Most diabetic patients manage their condition by using glucometers.

Glucometers measure the level of glucose in the bloodstream. During a potential hypoglycemic episode, if at all possible, ask the person if they have used their glucometer lately or encourage them to use it immediately. If the person is still cognizant but looks "out of it," you may have to assist in the process. A blood glucose value of less than 80 milligrams per deciliter can be considered a hypoglycemic episode. This kind of reading would prompt a swift glucose administration and, in worst-case scenarios, a trip to the emergency room.

7. What is the main idea of the passage?

A) Medical professionals should know what causes hypoglycemia and how to manage it.

B) Glucometers help patients with diabetes monitor their glucose levels.

C) Patients with diabetes can slip into a diabetic coma if they do not monitor their glucose levels.

D) Profuse sweating is one of the most telltale signs of a hypoglycemic episode.

8. What is the meaning of the word *administer* in the second paragraph?

A) adorn

B) give

C) revive

D) withdraw

9. Which of the following is NOT listed as a detail in the passage?

A) Glucometers help patients and medical professionals measure the level of glucose in the bloodstream.

B) Any blood glucose value that reads less than 80 milligrams per deciliter can be considered a hypoglycemic episode.

C) Only people with diabetes can become hypoglycemic.

D) Hypoglycemia literally means low (*hypo*) blood sugar (*glycemia*).

10. What is the author's primary purpose in writing this essay?

A) to inform health care workers and the public about the symptoms of hypoglycemia and how to respond to it

B) to persuade people to purchase more glucometers so that they can properly handle all hypoglycemic episodes

C) to dramatize a hypoglycemic episode so readers will know what to expect if they encounter a patient with diabetes who is undergoing one

D) to recount a time when a medical professional failed to properly respond to a hypoglycemic episode

11. Which of the following statements is a fact stated in the passage?

A) Profuse sweating is the number one sign that tells a medical professional a hypoglycemic episode has concluded.

B) Any blood glucose value that reads less than 80 milligrams per deciliter can be considered a hypoglycemic episode.

C) Most diabetic patients do not know how to monitor their own condition, so health care workers must help them.

D) Most personal glucometers are outdated, and medical professionals should purchase their own.

12. Which of the following statements can the reader infer from the passage?

A) Diabetic comas, which can be triggered by untreated episodes of hypoglycemia, can cause permanent brain damage.

B) Glucometers are too expensive for most diabetic patients to purchase, making cases of hypoglycemia frequent.

C) Medical professionals should ignore the personal perspectives of people experiencing hypoglycemic episodes.

D) Diabetes is a dangerous disease that cannot be managed properly.

The following passage refers to questions 13–18.

Communicating with any human being in crisis—whether that crisis is physical or emotional—is going to be more difficult than normal, everyday communication. Thus, emergency responders and medical practitioners, like many other social service providers, need to learn how to be sensitive in interpersonal communication. Here are some tips about how to hone your craft as a communicator while working with people in crisis. These tips can also be used for everyday communication.

First, it is essential that you are aware of cultural differences. In some cultures, direct eye contact can be unsettling or disrespectful. People from different cultures may have different comfort levels with personal space: some might find physical closeness comforting; others might find it threatening. Your body language speaks volumes. Be sure you are aware of the symbolic nature of your posture, hand motions, and gestures.

It is also important to enunciate your verbal statements and directions in a clear, relevant way. Use terminology and directions that a patient will understand, and avoid lofty medical jargon. Believe it or not, you also want to be honest with the person in crisis, even if the conditions are dire. Also explain, if possible, what you might do to help alleviate even the most drastic conditions so that the person feels supported. Lastly, and most importantly, be prepared to listen. Even if there is a language barrier, condition, or disability limiting your communication with the person in crisis, try to position yourself as an active listener. These tips will help you support people who need clarity and sensitivity.

13. What is the best summary of the passage?

   A) In some cultures, direct eye contact can be unsettling or disrespectful.

   B) Posture, hand motions, and gestures can symbolize respect or disrespect.

   C) Medical practitioners must learn to be sensitive with people who are in crisis.

   D) Medical practitioners should give clear directions and avoid using lofty medical jargon.

14. What is the author's primary purpose in writing this essay?

   A) to warn people about the dangers of disrespectful communication

   B) to persuade medical personnel to speak only when it is necessary

   C) to tell an interesting story about a paramedic who offended a patient

   D) to advise medical practitioners about communicating with patients in crisis

15. According to the passage, what is true about cultural differences?

   A) People from most cultures can recognize a thumbs-up gesture.

   B) In some cultures, people are uncomfortable with direct eye contact.

   C) When a crisis occurs, cultural differences usually disappear.

   D) No matter what someone's culture is, everyone needs a hug in a crisis.

16. Which of the following statements can be considered a statement of FACT according to the content offered in the paragraphs above?

   A) Most people cannot handle it if you look them in the eye and tell "dire" truths.

   B) Communicating with someone in crisis is more difficult than normal communication.

   C) The most important part of sensitive communication is establishing physical contact.

   D) Communicating with patients is not as important as dealing quickly with their injuries.

17. According to the passage, what do most people in crisis need?

   A) medical care
   B) psychological counseling
   C) cultural understanding
   D) sensitivity and clarity

18. What is the meaning of the phrase "speaks volumes" in the second paragraph?

   A) talks too much
   B) reads instructions
   C) communicates many things
   D) reads novels in several volumes

The following passage refers to questions 19–22.

Empathy is different from mimicry or sympathy—it is neither imitating someone else's emotions nor feeling concern for their suffering. Empathy is much more complex; it is the ability to actually share and comprehend the emotions of others.

Empathy takes on two major forms: cognitive empathy and affective, or emotional, empathy. Cognitive empathy is the ability to identify and understand the emotions, mental state, or perspective of others. Affective empathy is the ability to experience an emotional response to the emotions of others—either to feel what they are feeling or to have an appropriate emotional reaction, such as feeling sad when hearing about someone's bad news. Related to affective empathy is compassionate empathy, the ability to control your own emotions while helping others deal with theirs.

Empathy is crucial for being able to respond properly in social settings. People who suffer from some psychiatric conditions, such as autism spectrum disorder, may struggle with being empathetic. Conversely, some people with very strong cognitive empathy may abuse their social understanding as a means to take advantage of others. Most people, however, choose moments and contexts in which they are likely to relate to the emotions of others.

19. The reader can infer from the passage that the author believes empathy is

A) a primarily positive quality.

B) similar to autism spectrum disorder.

C) similar to mimicry or sympathy.

D) a good quality is some cases and a bad quality in others.

20. What is the author's primary purpose in writing these paragraphs?

A) to define empathy

B) to persuade readers to show more empathy

C) to advise readers about ways to appear empathetic

D) to show that empathy is a better quality than sympathy

21. Which qualities can readers infer might be most useful to a medical professional who responds to emergencies?

A) sympathy and mimicry

B) cognitive empathy

C) affective empathy

D) compassionate empathy

22. According to the passage, what is one negative use of empathy?

A) People who actually possess little or no empathy may fake this quality.

B) People who are empathetic may feel too much concern for others' suffering.

C) People with affective empathy may experience an emotional response to others' emotions.

D) People who are able to identify and understand others' emotions, mental state, or perspective may abuse this knowledge by taking advantage of others.

Writing

Directions: Read the passage, and then answer the questions that follow.

The following passage refers to questions 1–3.

(1) Have you ever devoured a tasty snow cone only to experience the agony of a "brain freeze"? (2) Have you ever wondered why or how that happens? (3) Well, scientists now believe they understand the mechanism of these so-called ice cream headaches.

(4) It begins with the icy temperature of the snow cone (or any cold food, or sometimes even exposure to cold air). (5) When a cold substance (delicious or otherwise) presses against the roof of your mouth, it causes blood vessels there to begin constricting, and your body starts to sense that something is awry. (6) In response, blood is pumped to the affected region to try to warm it up, causing rapid dilation of the same vessels. (7) This causes the neighboring trigeminal nerve to send rapid signals to your brain. (8) Because the trigeminal nerve also serves the face. (9) The brain misinterprets these signals as coming from your forehead.

(10) Regardless of the time spent wincing, the danger of the ice cream headache that certainly will not stop people for screaming for their favorite frozen treat in the future.

1. Which sentence in the second paragraph is missing an independent clause?

   A) sentence 5

   B) sentence 6

   C) sentence 7

   D) sentence 8

2. Which sentence contains an extra word?

   A) sentence 7, "to"

   B) sentence 8, "also"

   C) sentence 9, "as"

   D) sentence 10, "that"

3. Where is the best place to add this sentence?

   The duration of the pain varies from a few seconds up to about a minute.

   A) after sentence 3

   B) after sentence 4

   C) after sentence 9

   D) after sentence 10

The following passage refers to questions 4 and 5.

(1) The word *bacteria* typically conjures images of disease-inducing invaders that attack our immune systems. (2) However, recent research is changing that perception. (3) Plenty of scholarly articles point to the benefits of healthy bacteria that actually reinforce the immune system. (4) According to new research, the "microbiome"—that the resident bacteria in your digestive system—may impact your health in multiple ways. (5) Scientists who been studying microbial DNA now believe that internal bacteria can influence metabolism, mental health, and mood. (6) Some even suggest that imbalances in your digestive microbiome correlate with disorders like obesity and autoimmune diseases.

4. Which sentence contains an unnecessary word?

   A) sentence 1, "that"

   B) sentence 2, "that"

   C) sentence 3, "that"

   D) sentence 4, "that"

5. Which sentence has a verb error?

   A) sentence 3

   B) sentence 4

   C) sentence 5

   D) sentence 6

The following passage refers to questions 6 and 7.

(1) We all know how vital blood is for the human body—it transports oxygen from our lungs, removes waste from our organs, and protects our bodies from infections. (2) Blood feeds and stimulate the neurological processes of the nervous system. (3) It pumps waste products through the liver and kidneys of the excretory system. (4) It even releases antibodies so the immune system can help destroy potentially harmful microorganisms in the body. (5) Blood is one of the most versatile components of human life.

6. Where is the best place to add this sentence?

It plays an integral part in the processes of all other systems in the human body.

A) after sentence 1

B) after sentence 2

C) after sentence 3

D) after sentence 5

7. Which sentence has a verb error?

A) sentence 1

B) sentence 2

C) sentence 3

D) sentence 4

The following passage refers to questions 8–10.

(1) Across the globe, women are, on average, outliving their male counterparts. (2) Although this gender gap has shrunk over the last decade thanks to medical improvements and lifestyle changes, women are still expected to live four and a half years longer than men. (3) What are the reason for this trend? (4) The answer may lie in our sex hormones.

(5) Men are more likely to exhibit riskier behaviors than women, especially between the ages of fifteen and twenty-four, when testosterone production is at its peak. (6) Testosterone is correlated with aggressive and reckless behaviors that contribute to high mortality rates—think road rage, alcohol consumption, drug use, and smoking.

(7) Estrogen, on the other hand, seems to be correlated with cholesterol levels: an increase in estrogen is accompanied by a decrease in "bad" cholesterol, which may confer advantages by reducing the risk of heart attack and stroke.

(8) Of course, lifestyle and diet are also components of this difference in life expectancy. (9) Men are more likely to be involved in more physically dangerous jobs, such as manufacturing or construction. (10) They may be less likely to eat as many fruits and vegetables as their female counterparts. (11) And may be more likely to consume more red meat, including processed meat. (12) Better health decisions and better nutrition may eventually even the score in men's and women's life expectancy.

8. Which sentence contains a verb error?

A) sentence 1

B) sentence 2

C) sentence 3

D) sentence 4

9. Which sentence is missing a subject?

A) sentence 8

B) sentence 9

C) sentence 10

D) sentence 11

10. Where is the best place to add this sentence?

These types of meats have been linked to high cholesterol, hypertension, and cancer.

A) after sentence 7

B) after sentence 8

C) after sentence 11

D) after sentence 12

The following passage refers to questions 11–13.

(1) Autism is a psychiatric condition that exists along a spectrum ranging from mild to severe. (2) It affects communication, social interaction, and behavior. (3) People with severe cases of autism is likely to be unable to communicate verbally or nonverbally. (4) They do not initiate social interactions and may be unable to respond appropriately when spoken to. (5) They often engage in repetitive behaviors.

(6) On the other hand, people at the mild end of the spectrum may appear to have good social skills, making their condition less likely to be detected. (7) However, they may struggle with social situations. (8) They may have to be taught to make eye contact and how to engage in back-and-forth conversation with friends, peers, teachers, employers, and others. (9) And may have extremely focused interests and require routines to stay on an even keel.

(10) There is not a one-size-fits-all way to interact with people with autism spectrum disorder, so it is best for teachers, employers, coworkers, and friends to collaborate with these unique learners on a case-by-case basis.

11. Which sentence contains a verb error?

- **A)** sentence 1
- **B)** sentence 2
- **C)** sentence 3
- **D)** sentence 4

12. Which sentence is missing a subject?

- **A)** sentence 6
- **B)** sentence 7
- **C)** sentence 8
- **D)** sentence 9

13. Where is the best place to add this sentence?

People at this end of the spectrum need lifelong support.

- **A)** after sentence 4
- **B)** after sentence 5
- **C)** after sentence 6
- **D)** after sentence 7

The following passage refers to questions 14 and 15.

(1) A variety of environmental factors can inhibit the body's ability to naturally keep itself cool. (2) On the other hand, extremely dry heat may encourage people to push beyond their normal boundaries of exertion because they do not "feel" the heat as much as in humid environments. (3) Overexertion in either moist or dry heat forces the body to alter its heat-coping mechanisms, placing people at risk of experiencing heat cramps, heat exhaustion, or heat stroke. (4) These physiological responses to heat exposure can impair important bodily functions and can even result in death.

(5) Heat cramps occur when an excessive amount of water and salts are released from the body—in the form of sweat—in hot conditions. (6) Prolonged loss of water and salts will lead to muscle cramps, usually in the legs or abdomen. (7) Excessive loss of fluids and salts can also lead to heat exhaustion, a state in which a person experiences shallow breathing, an altered mental state, unresponsiveness, dizziness or faintness, and/or moist and cool skin. (8) These symptoms occur as a result of circulatory dysfunction. (9) The overexposure to heat combined with the loss of fluids disrupted normal blood flow.

14. Which sentence contains a verb error?

- **A)** sentence 6
- **B)** sentence 7
- **C)** sentence 8
- **D)** sentence 9

15. Where is the best place to add this sentence?

Humid conditions, for instance, mean that sweat evaporates slowly, reducing the body's ability to radiate heat.

A) after sentence 1

B) after sentence 2

C) after sentence 3

D) after sentence 4

The following passage refers to questions 16 and 17.

(1) Inflammation is one of the body's most vital forms of defense. (2) But can also be detrimental if it does not "turn off" or if it rushes to the aid of otherwise healthy tissue. (3) Inflammatory diseases like inflammatory bowel disease (IBD) or rheumatoid arthritis can have debilitating effects. (4) Chronic inflammation can cause pain, fatigue, gastrointestinal problems, and other symptoms. (5) Anti-inflammatory medications and certain steroids can lessen the inflammation and relieved some of the symptoms.

16. Which sentence is missing a subject?

A) sentence 1

B) sentence 2

C) sentence 3

D) sentence 4

17. Which sentence has a verb error?

A) sentence 2

B) sentence 3

C) sentence 4

D) sentence 5

The following passage refers to questions 18 and 19.

(1) Hormone feedback systems can involve steroid hormones. (2) For example, testosterone is a steroid hormone that influences male secondary sexual characteristics that develop during puberty. (3) Its level is influenced by the production of follicle-stimulating hormone (FSH) and luteinizing hormone (LH) in a negative feedback loop. (4) When testosterone reaches a certain level, it inhibits the production of FSH and LH. (5) As testosterone levels fall, FSH and LH begin to be released again, starting the cycle over. (6) A similar but more complex feedback loop occurs in women with FSH and LH stimulating the production of estrogen. (7) Resulting in the cycle of ovulation and menstruation.

18. Where is the best place to add this sentence?

The release of FSH and LH stimulates the production of testosterone.

A) after sentence 1

B) after sentence 2

C) after sentence 3

D) after sentence 4

19. Which sentence contains a grammar error?

A) sentence 4

B) sentence 5

C) sentence 6

D) sentence 7

The following passage refers to questions 20 and 21.

(1) In 2016, President Barack Obama's administration released its national dietary guidelines, which featured some changes from earlier versions. (2) While previous national guidelines focused on the dangers of cholesterol; the Obama administration's new guidelines highlighted the dangers of processed sugar. (3) According to the guidelines, sugar should account for no more than 10 percent of a healthy adult's total daily calories, or about 200 calories. (4)

Obama's guidelines warning against the dangers of "empty calories" such as those from soft drinks. (5) In particular, the guidelines called for an increased awareness of sugar consumption among men, who are disproportionately affected by excessive sugar intake. (6) They urged men to eat more vegetables and foods with fiber to help stave off health risks like heart disease, colon cancer, hypertension, stroke, and diabetes, some of which are directly correlated with the overconsumption of sugar.

20. Which sentence contains a punctuation error?

A) sentence 1

B) sentence 2

C) sentence 3

D) sentence 4

21. Which sentence contains a verb error?

A) sentence 3

B) sentence 4

C) sentence 5

D) sentence 6

Mathematics

Directions: Work the problem, and then choose the correct answer.

1. A pharmacy technician fills 13 prescriptions in 30 minutes. At that rate, how many prescriptions can he fill in a 7-hour shift?

   A) 91

   B) 45

   C) 182

   D) 208

2. A patient weighs 110 pounds. What is her weight in kilograms?

   A) 55 kg

   B) 50 kg

   C) 11 kg

   D) 20 kg

3. A patient has a condition that requires her to limit her fluid intake to 1800 milliliters per day. A family member brings her a bottle of water that contains 591 milliliters, and she drinks the whole bottle. How many milliliters of water can the patient ingest the rest of the day?

   A) 1391 ml

   B) 1209 ml

   C) 2391 ml

   D) 1309 ml

4. Andre welded together three pieces of metal pipe, measuring 26.5 inches, 18.9 inches, and 35.1 inches. How long was the welded pipe?

   A) 10.3 in

   B) 80.5 in

   C) 27.5 in

   D) 42.7 in

5. A doctor advises her prediabetic patient to decrease his sugar consumption by 25%. If he currently consumes 40 grams of sugar per day on average, how many grams of sugar per day should he have now?

   A) 10 g

   B) 16 g

   C) 24 g

   D) 30 g

6. In its first year of business, a small company lost $2100. The next year, the company recorded a profit of $11,200. What was the company's average profit over the two years?

   A) $5650

   B) $4550

   C) $9100

   D) $11,300

7. Bob's hospital bill is $1896. If Bob pays $158 per month, which expression represents his balance after x months?

   A) $158(1896 - x)$

   B) $158x + 1896$

   C) $1738x$

   D) $1896 - 158x$

8. The dosage for a certain medication is 2 milligrams per kilogram. What dosage should be given to a patient weighing 165 pounds?

   A) 150 mg

   B) 250 mg

   C) 132 mg

   D) 50 mg

9. The ratio of men to women in a nursing program is 2 to 7. If there are 72 men in the program, how many women are there?

A) 504 women

B) 21 women

C) 252 women

D) 210 women

10. A doctor has prescribed Norco 10/325, which contains 10 milligrams of hydrocodone and 325 milligrams of acetaminophen , to help control a patient's post-op pain. The warning on the prescription label cautions patients to limit their intake of acetaminophen to less than 3500 milligrams per day. How many tablets can the patient take while staying under the daily limit?

A) 9

B) 10

C) 11

D) 12

11. Chris makes $13.50 an hour. How much will he earn in a 7.5-hour day?

A) $101.25

B) $1012.50

C) $20.75

D) $91.00

12. How much alcohol by volume is in a 500 milliliter bottle of 70% isopropyl alcohol?

A) 35 ml

B) 50 ml

C) 400 ml

D) 350 ml

13. Rosie has $145. She needs to buy a new dishwasher that costs $520. How much will she need to save each week to be able to buy the dishwasher in five weeks?

A) $75

B) $80

C) $104

D) $133

14. The average high temperature in Paris, France, in July is 25°C. Convert the temperature to Fahrenheit.

A) 13°F

B) 43°F

C) 77°F

D) 57°F

15. The recommended dosage of a particular medication is 4 milliliters per 50 pounds of body weight. What is the recommended dosage for a person who weighs 175 pounds?

A) 25 ml

B) 140 ml

C) 14 ml

D) 28 ml

16. A medication's expiration date has passed. The label says it contains 600 milligrams of ibuprofen, but it has lost 125 milligrams of ibuprofen. How much ibuprofen is left in the tablet?

A) 475 mg

B) 525 mg

C) 425 mg

D) 125 mg

17. Dashawn is baking two desserts for Thanks-giving dinner. One recipe calls for $2\frac{1}{2}$ cups of flour and the other recipe calls for $1\frac{1}{3}$ cups of flour. If the flour canister had 8 cups of flour before he started baking, how much flour is left?

A) $4\frac{3}{5}$ c

B) $5\frac{5}{6}$ c

C) $4\frac{1}{6}$ c

D) $5\frac{2}{5}$ c

18. A hospital delivered 2213 babies last year, and 44% of those babies were boys. How many boys were born in that hospital last year? Round the answer to the nearest whole number.

A) 1239 boys

B) 1170 boys

C) 974 boys

D) 503 boys

19. If the average person drinks ten 8-ounce glasses of water each day, how many ounces of water will she drink in a week?

A) 80 oz

B) 700 oz

C) 560 oz

D) 70 oz

20. If one serving of milk contains 280 milligrams of calcium, how much calcium is in 1.5 servings?

A) 187 mg

B) 295 mg

C) 420 mg

D) 200 mg

21. Solve: $5(x + 3) - 12 = 43$

A) 8

B) 12

C) 9

D) 10

22. Normal body temperature is 98.6°F. Convert the temperature to Celsius.

A) 37°C

B) 54.8°C

C) 66.6°C

D) 47°C

23. Alice ran $3\frac{1}{2}$ miles on Monday, and she increased her distance by $\frac{1}{4}$ mile each day. What was her total distance from Monday to Friday?

A) $17\frac{1}{2}$ mi

B) 20 mi

C) $18\frac{1}{2}$ mi

D) 19 mi

24. An expired medication originally contained 500 milligrams of the active ingredient, but the content is now 150 milligrams. What percent of the active ingredient has been lost?

A) 30%

B) 70%

C) 35%

D) 50%

25. Jack missed 5% of 260 work days last year, some for illness and some for vacation. How many days did Jack work?

A) 13 days

B) 208 days

C) 247 days

D) 255 days

26. Fried's rule for computing an infant's dose of medication is:

$$\frac{\text{child's age in months} \times \text{adult dosage}}{150}$$

If the adult dose is 25 milligrams, how much should be given to a one-and-a-half-year-old child?

A) 3 mg

B) 6 mg

C) 4 mg

D) 5 mg

27. A carpenter is planning to add wood trim along three sides of a doorway. The sides of the doorway measure $7\frac{1}{2}$ feet, $2\frac{5}{8}$ feet, and $7\frac{1}{2}$ feet. How much wood trim is needed?

A) $16\frac{5}{8}$ ft

B) $17\frac{5}{8}$ ft

C) $16\frac{1}{2}$ ft

D) $17\frac{1}{2}$ ft

28. Kenna lost an average of 1.1 pounds per week for an entire year. How much weight did she lose? (Round to the nearest whole number.)

A) 47 lb

B) 53 lb

C) 46 lb

D) 58 lb

Science

Directions: Read the question, and then choose the most correct answer.

1. Which of the following types of cell carries hemoglobin in the blood?

   A) white blood cell

   B) red blood cell

   C) platelet

   D) T cell

2. The incus, stapes, and malleus play an important role in which sense?

   A) vision

   B) taste

   C) hearing

   D) smell

3. Which of the following is released when bone is broken down?

   A) phosphorous

   B) iron

   C) calcium

   D) zinc

4. Which chamber of the heart pumps deoxygenated blood to the lungs?

   A) right atrium

   B) right ventricle

   C) left atrium

   D) left ventricle

5. Which of the following is the network of capillaries in the kidneys where filtration begins?

   A) renal pelvis

   B) collecting ducts

   C) ureters

   D) glomerulus

6. A patient came to the emergency department complaining of severe lower back pain after a fall. Which vertebrae has the patient most likely injured?

   A) cervical

   B) thoracic

   C) cranial

   D) lumbar

7. Which of the following explains why people experience heartburn?

   A) The esophageal sphincter does not fully close.

   B) The epiglottis remains closed after swallowing.

   C) The stomach was unable to digest its contents.

   D) The pharynx pushes air into the esophagus.

8. A patient with a blocked cerebral artery is experiencing what?

   A) subdural hematoma

   B) myocardial infarction

   C) hemorrhagic stroke

   D) ischemic stroke

9. Which of the following is found in the blood in high levels as a result of muscle fatigue?

   A) ATP

   B) platelets

   C) lactic acid

   D) glucose

10. Which of the following is the largest and outermost part of the brain?

    A) pons
    B) cerebellum
    C) cerebrum
    D) thalamus

11. The hardening and narrowing of the arteries due to plaque buildup is known as

    A) gingivitis.
    B) atherosclerosis.
    C) thrombosis.
    D) melanoma.

12. What is the role of the liver in digestion?

    A) It produces the bile needed to digest fats.
    B) It stores bile produced by the gallbladder.
    C) It regulates feelings of hunger.
    D) It collects the waste that is the end product of digestion.

13. Which of the following hormones is released by the kidneys and helps regulate blood pressure?

    A) renin
    B) calcitriol
    C) cortisol
    D) oxytocin

14. Which of the following is a function of cerebrospinal fluid?

    A) It prevents the layers of the meninges from sticking together.
    B) It mixes with blood to nourish the brain.
    C) It removes waste products from the brain.
    D) It transmits signals to and from the brain.

15. A patient arrives in the emergency room complaining of shortness of breath. A blood test shows that her iron level is low. Which of the following will likely also be decreased?

    A) hemoglobin
    B) plasma
    C) white blood cells
    D) platelets

16. What substance does a Schwann cell secrete that increases the speed of signals traveling to and from neurons?

    A) myelin
    B) cerebrospinal fluid
    C) corpus callosum
    D) collagen

17. Which of the following structures begins the heartbeat by starting an electrical impulse in the right atrium?

    A) atrioventricular (AV) node
    B) sinoatrial (SA) node
    C) bundle of His
    D) mitral valve

18. Which of the following is a function of antibodies during an immune response?

    A) They store information for antibody production when the antigen reappears.
    B) They ingest the pathogen and destroy it.
    C) They produce an enzyme to coat and protect healthy cells.
    D) They bind to the antigen to neutralize pathogens.

19. A patient's blood pressure is 120/80. Which of the following numbers represents the arterial pressure when the ventricles are contracting?

A) 120

B) 80

C) 240

D) 40

20. Which of the following connects the ribs sternum?

A) costal cartilage

B) synovial joint

C) cardiac muscle

D) collagen fiber

o the

Answer Key

1. **D) is correct.** The primary purpose of the essay is to inform; its focus is the endocrine system's parts and functions. It is not persuasive or cautionary.

2. **D) is correct.** In the second paragraph, the author writes, "The endocrine system's function is to produce and distribute hormones."

3. **A) is correct.** The answer provides an adequate summary of the passage overall. The other choices only provide specific details from the passage.

4. **B) is correct.** The author writes, "Hormones are also released in humans in moments of fear or anxiety and can trigger the fight-or-flight response." There are no sentences supporting the other claims.

5. **A) is correct.** In the first paragraph, the author writes, "The pituitary gland serves as the 'master gland' of the endocrine system."

6. **A) is correct.** In the second paragraph, the author writes, "When the hormones reach other tissues, they catalyze certain chemical reactions, stimulating various processes or activities." The writer then goes on to describe those activities in detail, making it clear that the hormones caused those events to occur.

7. **A) is correct.** The passage is about how important it is for medical professionals to understand hypoglycemia, especially when it comes to patients who have diabetes. The other answer choices are details from the passage.

8. **B) is correct.** In the second paragraph, the author writes, "You will likely need to help administer glucose to them as soon as possible." In this case, *administer* means to give glucose to a patient.

9. **C) is correct.** This detail is not found in the passage. The passage strongly focuses on patients with diabetes, but it does not state that only those patients are affected by hypoglycemia.

10. **A) is correct.** The text is informative, not persuasive or dramatic. It does not recount a specific event, but simply informs the audience of potential general scenarios.

11. **B) is correct.** In the third paragraph, the author writes, "A blood glucose value of less than 80 milligrams per deciliter can be considered a hypoglycemic episode."

12. **A) is correct.** In the second paragraph, the author states, "When a diabetic patient's blood sugar plummets, their mental state becomes altered. This can lead to unconsciousness or, in more severe cases, a diabetic coma and/or brain damage." The reader can infer from this information that diabetic comas *could* cause *permanent* brain damage.

13. **C) is correct.** The answer provides an adequate summary of the passage overall. The other choices only provide specific details from the passage.

14. **D) is correct.** The primary purpose of the essay is to advise; its focus is communication with patients in crisis. It is not persuasive or cautionary, and it does not tell a story.

15. **B) is correct.** The author writes, "In some cultures, direct eye contact can be unsettling or disrespectful." There are no sentences supporting the other claims.

16. **B) is correct.** In the first paragraph, the author writes, "Communicating with any human being in crisis—whether that crisis is physical or emotional—is going to be more difficult than normal, everyday communication."

17. **D) is correct.** In the last sentence, the author writes, "These tips will help you support people who need clarity and sensitivity."

18. **C) is correct.** In the second paragraph, the author writes, "Your body language speaks volumes." The writer then goes on to detail ways that body language can convey messages (with "posture, hand motions, and gestures").

19. **A) is correct.** In the last paragraph, the author states, "Empathy is crucial for being able to respond properly in social settings." The reader can infer from this information that empathy is a positive quality that people need in order to treat others in a socially acceptable manner.

20. **A) is correct.** The primary purpose of the essay is to inform; its focus is on the definition of empathy. It is not persuasive or advisory. The author does not set out to show that one quality is better than another.

21. **D) is correct.** In the second paragraph, the author defines compassionate empathy as "the ability to control your own emotions while helping others deal with theirs." Readers can infer that this kind of empathy would be useful to medical professionals who have to remain calm in emergencies (when patients and bystanders are often upset).

22. **D) is correct.** In the last paragraph the author writes, "Some people with very strong cognitive empathy may abuse their social understanding as a means to take advantage of others." Earlier the author defines "cognitive empathy" as "the ability to identify and understand the emotions, mental state, or perspective of others."

WRITING

1. **D) is correct.** Sentence 8 is actually a dependent clause.

2. **D) is correct.** Sentence 10 contains an unnecessary word, "that": "the danger of the ice cream headache *that* will certainly not stop people..."

3. **C) is correct.** This sentence explains the "signals" referred to in sentence 9 as "pain." Sentence 10 refers to "wincing," providing a clue that more context about pain is needed. This sentence should be placed after sentence 9.

4. **D) is correct.** Sentence 4 has an unnecessary occurrence of the word *that*: "that the resident bacteria."

5. **C) is correct.** Sentence 5 contains an error in conjugation: "Scientists who been studying." It should be corrected as: "Scientists who *have* been studying."

6. **A) is correct.** This sentence introduces the idea that blood is important for all body systems. The word "other" suggests that more body systems will be discussed. It should be placed after sentence 1 to introduce the ideas in sentences 2, 3, and 4, which refer to specific body systems.

7. **B) is correct.** Sentence 2 contains a verb error. The verb "stimulate" should be the singular "stimulates" to agree with the subject "Blood."

8. **C) is correct.** Sentence 3 contains a verb error: the verb "are" should be the singular "is" to agree with its singular subject, "reason."

9. **D) is correct.** Sentence 11 has no subject: it needs a word like "they" or "men" to be complete.

10. **C) is correct.** Sentence 11 specifically refers to "red meat" and "processed meat." This new sentence should be placed immediately after to provide more information about the consequences of consuming red and processed meat.

11. **C) is correct.** Sentence 3 contains a verb error. The singular verb "is" should be replaced with the plural verb "are" to agree with its plural subject, "People."

12. **D) is correct.** Sentence 9 is missing a subject; it needs a pronoun like "they" to be complete.

13. **B) is correct.** Sentence 5 completes a paragraph about severe cases of autism, and sentence 6 opens a new paragraph describing the "mild end of the spectrum." Placing this new sentence, which also mentions a "spectrum," after sentence 5 is a good way to complete the first paragraph, clarify the needs of people with more severe cases of autism, and transition to the new paragraph.

14. **D) is correct.** In sentence 9, the verb "disrupted" is conjugated incorrectly in the simple past tense. The other verbs in this paragraph are conjugated in the present tense, so it should be too ("disrupts").

15. **A) is correct.** This sentence provides more information about the "environmental factors" mentioned in sentence 1. It also leads to the transition phrase "on the other hand" beginning sentence 3, which then goes on to introduce "extremely dry heat," which is a counter example to the "humid conditions" discussed in the new sentence.

16. **B) is correct.** Sentence 2 requires a subject like the pronoun "it" or the word "inflammation" to be complete.

17. **D) is correct.** In sentence 5, the participle "relieved" should be conjugated "relieve."

18. **C) is correct.** FSH and LH are first mentioned in sentence 3, where the acronyms are spelled out. That is a good clue that the new sentence should be placed after sentence 3, where the terms have been introduced and the acronyms explained. The context and discussion of the action of testosterone suggests the new sentence should precede sentence 4.

19. **D) is correct.** Sentence 7 is not an independent clause; it lacks a subject or an active verb.

20. **B) is correct.** Sentence 2 contains a semicolon that incorrectly connects a dependent clause ("While previous national guidelines focused on the dangers of cholesterol") with an independent clause ("the Obama administration's new guidelines highlighted the dangers of processed sugar.") Semicolons should be used to join two independent clauses.

21. **B) is correct.** In sentence 4, the verb "warning" should be conjugated "warned" to match the subject "guidelines" and be written in the simple past tense to match verbs in the surrounding sentences.

MATHEMATICS

1. **C) is correct.**

   30 minutes = 0.5 hour

   $\frac{13}{0.5} = \frac{x}{7}$

   $0.5x = 91$

   x = 182

2. **B) is correct.**

   $110 \text{ lb} \times \frac{1 \text{ kg}}{2.2 \text{ lb}} \approx \textbf{50 kg}$

3. **B) is correct.**

   1800 − 591 = **1209**

4. **B) is correct.**

   26.5 + 18.9 + 35.1 = **80.5**

5. **D) is correct.**

   part = whole × percent

   40 × 0.25 = 10

   40 − 10 = **30**

6. **B) is correct.**

   −2100 + 11,200 = $9100

   $9100 ÷ 2 = **$4550**

7. **D) is correct.**

   If Bob pays $158 per month, the amount he has paid on his bill would be 158 times the number of months, x. Bob's balance will be decreased by the amount he has paid.

8. **A) is correct.**

   $\frac{2 \text{ mg}}{\text{kg}} \times \frac{1 \text{ kg}}{2.2 \text{ lb}} \times 165 \text{ lb} = \textbf{150 mg}$

9. **C) is correct.**

   $\frac{2}{7} = \frac{72}{x}$

   $2x = 504$

   x = 252

10. **B) is correct.**

    3500 ÷ 325 ≈ 10.8, so **10 tablets will stay under the limit**.

11. **A) is correct.**

    $13.50 × 7.5 = **$101.25**

12. **D) is correct.**

    part = whole × percent

    500 × 0.70 = **350**

13. **A) is correct.**

    Let x equal the amount of money Rosie needs to save each week.

    145 + 5x = 520

    5x = 375

    x = 75

14. **C) is correct.**

    F = 1.8C + 32

    F = 1.8(25) + 32

    F = 77°

15. **C) is correct.**

    $\frac{4}{50} = \frac{x}{175}$

    $50x = 700$

    x = 14

16. **A) is correct.**
    $600 - 125 = \mathbf{475}$

17. **C) is correct.**
    $2\frac{1}{2} + 1\frac{1}{3} = 2\frac{3}{6} + 1\frac{2}{6} = 3\frac{5}{6}$
    $8 - 3\frac{5}{6} = \frac{48}{6} - \frac{23}{6} = \frac{25}{6} = \mathbf{4\frac{1}{6}}$

18. **C) is correct.**
    part = whole × percent
    $2213 \times 0.44 = 973.72 \approx \mathbf{974}$

19. **C) is correct.**
    1 week = 7 days
    $10 \times 8 \times 7 = \mathbf{560}$

20. **C) is correct.**
    $\frac{1}{280} = \frac{1.5}{x}$
    $\mathbf{x = 420}$

21. **A) is correct.**
    $5(x + 3) - 12 = 43$
    $5x + 15 - 12 = 43$
    $5x + 3 = 43$
    $5x = 40$
    $\mathbf{x = 8}$

22. **A) is correct.**
    $C = \frac{5}{9}(F - 32)$

    $C = \frac{5}{9}(98.6 - 32)$
    $C = \frac{5}{9}(66.6) = \mathbf{37°}$

23. **B) is correct.**
    $3\frac{2}{4} + 3\frac{3}{4} + 4 + 4\frac{1}{4} + 4\frac{2}{4} = 18\frac{8}{4} = 18 + 2 = \mathbf{20}$

24. **B) is correct.**
    $500 - 150 = 350$ mg lost
    $\text{percent} = \frac{\text{part}}{\text{whole}}$
    $\frac{350}{500} = 0.7 = \mathbf{70\%}$

25. **C) is correct.**
    part = whole × percent
    $260 \times 0.05 = 13$
    $260 - 13 = \mathbf{247}$

26. **A) is correct.**
    $1\frac{1}{2}$ years = 18 months
    $\frac{18 \times 25}{150} = \mathbf{3}$

27. **B) is correct.**
    $7\frac{4}{8} + 2\frac{5}{8} + 7\frac{4}{8} = 16\frac{13}{8} = 16 + 1\frac{5}{8} = \mathbf{17\frac{5}{8}}$

28. **D) is correct.**
    1 year = 52 weeks
    $1.1 \times 52 = 57.5 \approx \mathbf{58}$

SCIENCE

1. **B) is correct.** Red blood cells contain hemoglobin, which has an iron component that transports oxygen. Hemoglobin also makes the red blood cells appear red in color.

2. **C) is correct.** The incus, stapes, and malleus are bones connected to the skull inside the ear. They play an important role in the sense of hearing.

3. **C) is correct.** Calcium is released as bones are degraded, helping balance the calcium level in the body.

4. **B) is correct.** Deoxygenated blood in the heart is delivered to the lungs for gas exchange from the right ventricle.

5. **D) is correct.** The glomerulus is a network of capillaries that begins the filtration process by filtering blood plasma, the result of which is then excreted as urine.

6. **D) is correct.** Lumbar vertebrae are also called the lower back vertebrae.

7. **A) is correct.** The esophagus has a sphincter that should close as food enters the stomach. If it does not fully close, it permits backflow of the stomach contents to the esophagus, causing heartburn.

8. **D) is correct.** The patient is having an ischemic stroke. An ischemic stroke is caused by a blockage of an artery supplying blood to the brain.

9. **C) is correct.** Lactic acid is elevated in the blood when prolonged muscle contraction causes muscle fatigue.

10. **C) is correct.** The cerebrum is the largest and outermost part of the brain.

11. **B) is correct.** Atherosclerosis occurs when arteries are hardened and/or narrowed due to the deposition of fatty plaques on the inner walls.

12. **A) is correct.** The liver produces bile, which is needed for the digestion of fats.

13. **A) is correct.** Renin is released by the kidneys and plays a role in regulating blood pressure.

14. **C) is correct.** Cerebrospinal fluid absorbs waste products from the brain, allowing them to be transferred into the bloodstream.

15. **A) is correct.** Hemoglobin is rich in iron, which allows it to transport oxygen to cells. Thus, a low iron level will likely correspond to a low hemoglobin level.

16. **A) is correct.** Schwann cells secrete myelin, which forms a sheath around the neuron and allows the electrical signal to travel faster.

17. **B) is correct.** The sinoatrial (SA) node starts the electrical conduction pathway for the heart by producing a regular impulse that causes the atria to contract. On an ECG this is reflected by the P wave.

18. **D) is correct.** Antibodies bind to the antigen on the pathogen, neutralizing the pathogen and attracting phagocytes.

19. **A) is correct.** The blood pressure is read as the systolic pressure over the diastolic pressure. During systole, the ventricles are contracting, and blood is being pumped out into the body. The systolic pressure measurement (here, 120), is thus the pressure in the arteries while the ventricles are contracting.

20. **A) is correct.** Costal cartilage connects the ribs to the sternum.

TO ACCESS YOUR SECOND KNAT PRACTICE TEST, FOLLOW THE LINK BELOW:

http://ascenciatestprep.com/knat-online-resources